The
Weight
Loss Triad

A Comprehensive Guide to Lasting Weight Loss

Dr. Thomas L Halton

Published by
Fitness Plus

First Edition

Published by Fitness Plus
Boston, MA

ISBN 978-0-615-22709-2

Table of Contents

Disclaimer

This book is intended for informational and educational purposes only. It is not meant to provide counseling, nor to provide medical advice. Always be sure to consult with your physician before starting any exercise program.

Chapter 1

Introduction To The Weight Loss Triad

I realize that this is probably the 10,000[th] book on weight loss that has been written in the past 50 years. If you have struggled with weight in your life, it is likely the 10th or 20th book that you have read on the subject. I truly believe that this could be your last.

Before we get started, I want you to get one thing straight. Weight loss is not easy. This program is not a quick fix. This book is not about following my "revolutionary program" and losing 10 pounds in a week. The sooner you understand this, the sooner you will realize that attaining your weight and health goals will take discipline and sacrifice and time. But the benefits are there. You will be repaid many fold for your effort, trust me. I envision this book as being for those who have tried a lot of the "miracle" diets and quick weight loss schemes and now realize that they just don't work. I envision this book being for those who want to know a little about the science of how their body gains and loses weight. I envision this book as being for those who want to know the real truth about how to lose weight safely, effectively and permanently.

It is also important to understand that changes in diet and exercise to lose weight are not temporary solutions that you apply for 3 months and then go back to your old habits. No way! My goal is to help my clients maintain diet and exercise habits for the rest of their lives. It is true that during the weight loss phase, the program is more strict than during weight maintenance, but a healthy weight and a healthy body require continued effort. If you can't accept this, this is certainly not the book for you. But unfortunately, you better learn to accept this because that is the way it is.

I have been helping people lose weight for over 10 years. The original motivation behind this book was to provide my clients with a workbook that would emphasize, in writing, what they need to be focusing on in order to reach their goals. I normally start my first meeting with a client by telling them a little about myself and my background. Since the format of this short book will loosely resemble a consultation with me, here goes.

My name is Dr. Thomas L. Halton and I grew up in Long Island, NY. After graduating college and giving law school a try (I lasted one semester-it clearly wasn't the career for me) I realized that a major passion of mine was to study exercise and diet and help people to live healthier and longer lives by applying what I had learned.

In 1995, I passed the American Council on Exercise Personal Trainer Exam and started working at a gym in Long Island. Shortly thereafter, I founded a small personal training company called Fitness Plus. In this business, I would enter a client's home and counsel them on exercise, usually with the goal of weight loss. It did not take me long to realize that this was the job for me. Although I had a good training background, it dawned on me that exercise really wasn't the whole answer to the weight loss problem. I needed to learn more about diet. I promptly began preparing for ACE's Lifestyle and Weight Management Counselor certifying examination and passed that in 1997. I also began reading everything I could about nutrition and weight loss; Atkins, The Zone, Sugar Busters, Protein Power. I read them all, many 2 or 3 times. I entered a Masters program in Exercise Science at Queens College in NY. After graduating from that program in 1999, I entered a Masters program in Human Nutrition at the University of Bridgeport, Connecticut.

After graduating that program, I sat for the American College of Nutrition Certified Nutrition Specialist examination. This certification, along with my Masters degrees and experience would allow me to become a Licensed Nutritionist. I loved all of this learning. Nutrition and exercise physiology are two fields that are very exciting. Both are young sciences and are therefore constantly changing. I wanted to learn more. In 2001, I began my biggest academic challenge to date; I entered Harvard University's doctoral program in Nutritional Epidemiology (the study of how nutrition affects disease) and finally graduated in 2006. Since then I've opened up a clinical nutrition counseling and personal training practice in Boston, MA, taught grad school part time at Simmons College in Boston and work part time as a Research Consultant for The Cooper Institute in Dallas, Texas.

So what did I learn from all of these degrees, certifications and experience? Well, that is the subject of this book. What you are holding in your hand is everything you need to know in order to lose weight effectively and permanently. A percentage of this knowledge is academic and based on research I learned or conducted along the way. On the other hand, a good amount is more "practical"; things I picked up in the past 10+ years helping people to lose weight in the real world.

At this point in the initial interview, I let the client know that they are about to receive an overwhelming amount of information. Most of which will require serious lifestyle changes that are not easy at first. I tell them that I am about to explain everything that they can do to lose weight the fastest, healthiest and most permanent way.

I don't expect them to immediately follow every principle perfectly. That is not really possible. I also tell them that I'm giving them the gold standard and that they will still lose weight with the silver or bronze standard, just a bit more slowly.

I have had a few rare clients that were able to incorporate just about everything right away, and let me say, they get amazing results. Most of my successful clients, however, focused on one area at a time. In the first few weeks they worked on resistance training and then focused on cardiovascular exercise and finally diet and lifestyle issues. This took place over a period of weeks and/or months. I think this is a great way to break down the program into smaller pieces that are easier to focus on.

Losing weight is a very personal thing and everyone has their own strengths and weaknesses that need to be worked with. Also, the path to weight loss is rarely a straight line. There are peaks and valleys. There will be times that you feel it's a snap and the pounds are rolling off. Then there will be times when the scale doesn't budge or you've relapsed a bit and the situation seems hopeless. This is all normal; expect it, but know this; I have never met a person in all of my years that wasn't able to lose weight with these changes. Everyone who follows these guidelines can make significant and permanent changes to their bodies. Of course, we can't all become Brad Pitt or Cameron Diaz. Our genes will have a say in that, but we all can achieve a healthier body weight, all the while increasing our energy and decreasing the risk of today's most deadly diseases.

I guess now would be a good time to explain the major concept and the name of this book; The Weight Loss Triad. A triad is simply a group of 3. Three is a very important number for those of you trying to lose weight. Three is the number of areas that need attention if your goal is permanent weight loss. More specifically the three areas are; 1) Diet 2) Cardiovascular exercise and 3) Resistance training.

The goal of the dietary component is to ensure a stable blood sugar. Humans were designed to have a stable blood sugar and most of the foods put on this Earth for us promote blood sugar stability. However, we have changed our food supply by processing and refining foods to the point that they barely resemble the foods we were intended to eat. Getting back to a stable blood sugar will decrease cravings and set your body up for fat burning instead of fat storage.

The goal of the cardiovascular exercise program is, quite simply, to burn calories. Obviously, this will help reduce stores of body fat. The goal of the resistance training program is two-fold. As we age, we start to lose muscle. Muscle is a metabolically active tissue which means that it takes a lot of calories to maintain muscle. The first goal of the weight training component is to not only stop this loss of lean tissue, but to add to it so you burn more calories everyday, just by breathing!

The second reason for resistance training during weight loss has to do with the human body defense mechanism to hold on to body fat. When you lose weight, your body gets nervous and wants to protect fat reserves for the future. Therefore, it will give up a bit of fat but after a point will start to burn muscle in addition to fat. So a person goes on a commercial weight loss plan and loses 10 pounds without re-sistance training. Little do they know that half of that weight loss was fat and the other half was muscle. So 5 lbs of muscle that was previously burning 250 calories per day is now ancient history.

Because of this drop in metabolism, the dieter hits a brick wall and stops losing weight. Since they are no longer losing weight, they stop their diet and begin to eat as they used to. They quickly gain back the 10 lbs they lost plus more because their metabolism is now operating with 5 lbs less muscle. This sequence is often repeated several times and is largely responsible for the yo-yo dieting syndrome everyone seems to be talking about. Resistance training helps to lessen this break-down of muscle with weight loss so more of the weight you lose will be fat. This results in permanent weight loss instead of yo-yo dieting.

It is easy to think of these 3 areas as a pyramid.

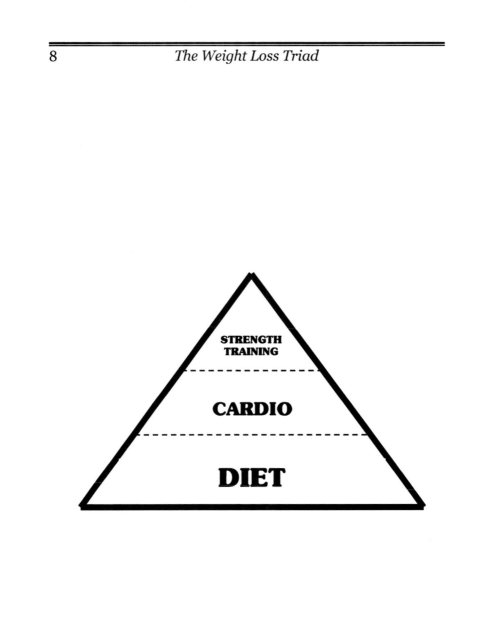

You may be familiar with the USDA Food Guide Pyramid or the Mediterranean Diet Pyramid. This weight loss pyramid is based on a similar principle. The most important part is the base; in this case diet. The next most important part is cardiovascular exercise and the third most important aspect of the program is resistance or strength training. This is a simple and quick way to show you how you should prioritize the different components of this program. In my experience, for those trying to lose weight, 50% of their results will come from dietary change, 30% from the cardiovascular exercise component and 20% from resistance training. Having said this, all three components are necessary to maximize fat loss. The pyramid is a rough guide to let you know how you should divide your valuable time and energy. If you want to lose weight, you should not spend your 6 weekly exercise sessions only lifting weights.

In the remainder of this book, I'll take you through each of these components in detail and teach you just about everything that I know in order to help you attain your weight loss goals in a safe and efficient manner. Along the way we'll accomplish other goals that may or not be important to you, such as increasing your energy, reducing the effects of stress, improving your sleeping habits, reducing the risk of heart disease, stroke, diabetes and cancer, boosting your immune system, decreasing the risk of osteoporosis, decreasing symptoms of anxiety and depression and boosting that all important self confidence. When I start with a new client, I really feel as though we are going on a mission together. There will be ups and downs, good times and bad but the goal is attainable. My job is to light a flame under you and hope it catches. Because once you realize the benefits of living the way I'm about to show you, you'll never want to go back. Are you ready? Are you psyched? Let's get to it.

ACTION STEPS FOR THIS CHAPTER

1) Realize mentally that weight loss is not quick or easy.

2) Realize that changes in diet and exercise habits need to be permanent for weight loss to be permanent.

3) Pace yourself with the lifestyle changes you will soon learn. Don't expect to change everything overnight. Chip away at it and try to get a little better each week.

4) Understand that when it comes to weight loss, 50% of your results will come from your dietary changes, 30% from your cardiovascular exercise habits and 20% from your resistance training program. Prioritize accordingly.

Introduction To Diet Plan

As mentioned previously, your diet is the most important component of your weight loss program and will have the biggest impact on your success or failure. So, now it's time to find out how to eat for success! The foods we eat can be broken down into 3 basic categories called macronutrients; they are protein, fat and carbohydrate. Although most foods contain all 3 of these macronutrients, one is usually represented much more than the others. In this section of the book, I will briefly explain the function of each of these macronutrients, and provide guidance on how to choose the best foods to help you lose weight and improve your health. At the end, we'll put it all together. I'll show you sample meal plans that will help you tailor this way of eating to your own personal preferences.

Now would be a good time to describe my own personal nutrition philosophy. I guess I am what you'd call an "evolutionary" nutritionist. I believe that

Mother Nature knows a lot more about what we should be eating than anyone or anything else. Certain foods were put on this Earth for us to consume while our internal systems were evolving. Man came along and started refining and processing foods and messed up this general formula for good health. If you look at the diet of the typical American, 70-80% of the foods consumed are no longer in their natural form. The major problem with this pertains to the maintenance of a steady blood sugar. The foods put on this Earth for us to consume, for the most part, have a very easy effect on our blood sugar. When we eat them, our blood glucose level rises gradually and we release a small amount of insulin to lower it back down. This is the way it should be. However, when we eat processed, refined carbohydrates, our blood glucose levels rise sharply and we need to release a very large amount of insulin to handle this peak.

This is where we run into problems. These large swings in blood sugar and insulin levels have a variety of negative effects. For starters, high insulin levels drive blood glucose below baseline and cause an increase in hunger. This will result in overeating and weight gain. There is also evidence that higher insulin levels may actually promote fat storage and inhibit the usage of lipoprotein lipase (an enzyme that tells our body to burn fat). This combination of increased hunger and enhanced fat deposition is a major concern for those looking to lose weight.

How can these swings in blood sugar be prevented? There are basically 2 strategies to ensure a stable blood sugar. 1) Choose carbohydrates that are easy on the blood sugar. These carbohydrates have what is known as a low glycemic load, which we will learn about later. 2) Every time you eat, combine a fat containing food, a protein containing food and a carbohydrate containing food. The addition of fat and protein to a carbohydrate slows the entry of that carbohydrate into the blood stream.

The human body contains macronutrient specific digestive enzymes. There are enzymes that just digest fat, enzymes that just digest protein and enzymes that just digest carbohydrate. For example, when you eat a plain bagel for breakfast, the carbohydrate digesting enzymes have direct access to the carbohydrate and convert it to blood sugar at a very fast rate causing a spike in blood glucose. Now if you ate that same bagel with some lox (protein) and cream cheese (fat), the protein, fat and carbohydrate would mix up in your stomach. The carbohydrate digesting enzymes would have to work around the fat and protein, which takes time, and therefore the carbohydrate would be digested much more slowly resulting in a lower peak glucose and insulin level.

Probably the most important thing to remember about this diet is Rule #1: Make sure you include some protein, some fat and some carbohydrate at every meal. This is pivotal to maintaining a steady blood sugar.

We'll get into the details in the next few chapters but for now just try to grasp this concept.

In the next part of our journey, we'll go through each of these three macronutrients, learn a bit about their functions and then find out which to focus on and which to avoid. We'll list the best choices for fat, protein and carbohydrate and then every time you eat, you will simply pick one food from the carbohydrate list, one from the fat list and one from the protein list. We'll then get into some meal planning and portions sizes and then you'll be all set on diet.

Chapter 2

Protein: The Overlooked Macronutrient

Protein is a great macronutrient to start with because most people already know what foods are high in protein and almost all of these foods are permitted. Eating enough protein is of paramount importance to the maintenance of optimal health. Aside from water, protein forms the major portion of a lean human body, just about 16 percent of body weight.

Some of the major functions of protein include;

1) <u>The formation of vital body compounds</u>. Each and every cell contains protein. All of the following are made primarily of protein; muscle, enzymes, lipoproteins, connective tissue, clotting factors, immune factors, a wide variety of hormones as well as the supporting structure inside bones. Most of these vital components are in a constant state of breakdown, reconstruction and repair. If a person doesn't eat enough protein, over many weeks and months, the protein repairing and rebuilding slows down. Eventually skeletal

muscle, the heart, the liver and other organs will decrease in size or amount to compensate; only your brain will resist this breakdown.

2) <u>Maintaining acid/base balance</u>.

3) <u>Ensuring fluid balance</u>.

4) <u>Immune function</u>. Proteins contribute vital parts of the cells used by the immune system.

5) <u>Protein can provide the body with a ready source of energy</u>. In general, protein contributes less than 5% of the body's total energy need.

6) <u>Formation of glucose</u>. During times of inadequate carbohydrate intake, our body has the ability to make glucose, a major cellular fuel, out of amino acids from proteins.

Now here is the take home message of this chapter; MAKE SURE YOU EAT SOME PROTEIN AT EVERY SINGLE MEAL. Protein slows the entry of carbohydrate into the blood stream. Remember, the fundamental philosophy behind this style of eating is the maintenance of a steady blood sugar, as nature intended. The inclusion of protein with every meal can help you maintain this steady blood sugar as well as provide a few other benefits.

For example, there is evidence that those who consume higher amounts of protein at a meal have a greater sense of fullness and tend to eat fewer calories at subsequent meals. I have found this to be quite true in my practice. My clients' hunger tends to decrease with the addition of protein at each meal. There is also strong evidence that protein has a higher dietary thermogenesis than fat or carbohydrate, which means that in order for your body to break down and use the protein you eat, you have to burn more calories than you do for fat or carbohydrates. While this difference is relatively small, these extra calories do add up over weeks and months.

I want to make it clear that I'm not advocating a very high protein diet here. Currently in the United States, we consume about 15% of our calories as protein. I don't want you eating 40 or 50% of your calories as protein. I do not think that is healthy and it may even be harmful to the kidneys of susceptible individuals. On the other hand, raising the percent of protein from 15% to 20-25% is a good idea for those trying to lose weight, particularly if that additional 5-10% increase in protein comes at the expense of refined carbohydrate. I also feel that this is a safe level of protein intake for healthy individuals. If you have certain medical conditions, particularly those influencing the kidneys, you will want to check with your doctor before increasing your level of protein intake.

So what are sources of protein and which should you choose? I've placed the dietary proteins into 3 categories. Best Choices, OK Choices and Those To Avoid. Your best choices are like a green traffic light; you can eat these selections regularly without any real concern about negative effects. The OK choices are like a yellow traffic light. When entering an intersection, if the light is yellow, you're probably OK to pass through but it may be a safer bet to wait for a green light. These foods will be mired in some recent controversy as to their health and/or weight loss effects and taken in moderation will likely not do much harm. Finally we have the choices to avoid; your red stop light. These are foods that will have a definite negative impact on your health and/or your ability to lose weight. Stopping in front of these foods will help you avoid a nutritional car wreck. So here goes for protein;

Best Choices*

Chicken w/o skin	Monkfish
Turkey w/o skin	Flounder
Lean Ham	Other Fish
Pork	Egg Whites
Lobster	Black Beans
Crab	Pink Beans
Scallops	Navy Beans
Clams	Chick Peas
Mussels	Lentils
Salmon	Other Beans
Scrod	Soy Protein
Chilean Sea Bass	

Can be consumed every day. These sources of protein are low in saturated fat and should form the core of your protein choices.

OK Choices*

Skim Milk	Filet Mignon
Low-fat Cottage Cheese	Lean Ground Beef
Low-fat Cheese	Lean Roast Beef
Low-fat Plain Yogurt	Shrimp
Whole Eggs	Tuna

Can have several times a week. These choices are pretty good but something about them makes me hesitate to recommend them for every day service. For example: whole eggs and shrimp are high in cholesterol, red meat when cooked may form harmful substances called nitrosamines that may cause cancer, dairy has a variety of problems which is discussed in the next section.

<u>Strictly Limit*</u>

Whole Milk	Pastrami
Whole Cottage Cheese	Bologna
Whole Yogurt	Sausage
Whole Cheese	Hot Dogs
Hamburger	Bacon
Steak	Other Fatty Cold
Salami	Cuts
Pepperoni	

These are foods that are known to adversely affect your health due to excessive saturated fat or the addition of nitrates or other harmful food additives.

A Note About Dairy

There has been some recent controversy concerning the necessity of dairy products in our diet. A lot of nutritionists recommend dairy as a source of both protein and calcium. I have some serious questions about whether this is such a good idea. To start with, I always view the diet from an evolutionary standpoint. In other words, what foods were put on this earth for man and woman to consume? Were we really meant to consume large amounts of dairy products?

Our digestive systems evolved over 100's and 1000's of years on the foods that were put here for us by Mother Nature, God or whatever you are comfortable with. If you take a look at nature, no animals consume milk after the age of about 6 months to a year and no animal drinks another species' milk; ever! So I have my doubts about the large number of servings of dairy recommended in the Food Guide Pyramid. Add to this the fact that many adults lack the enzyme lactase that breaks down milk sugar and the question becomes even more complicated. Another concern is the addition of growth hormone and antibiotics to the dairy supply. These are not great for you!

For the other side of the story, the bone health of my clients is of vital concern to me. There is an epidemic of osteoporosis in this country, mostly among women. Although the research goes back and forth on whether dairy intake decreases incidence of osteoporotic fracture, I'm still hesitant to totally eliminate dairy from my clients diet. I didn't want to get off track here, I just wanted to explain why dairy products did not make my best choice list for protein. I would probably say it is fine to have one serving of dairy most days of the week, but not more than that. Remember, physical activity is one of the very best ways to prevent osteoporosis. On this program you'll get plenty of that, trust me!

A Note About Fish

Fish are an excellent source of protein and omega 3 fatty acids (which are showing to have a multitude of health benefits). You may have been reading in the paper about mercury toxicity in our fish supply. This is a legitimate concern, particularly for women who are pregnant or trying to become pregnant. While mercury toxicity can cause a variety of symptoms in humans, it is particularly harmful to developing fetuses. Specifically, it can cause a decreased neurological development.

Mercury from industry and other sources accumulate in the tissue of fish dwelling in polluted regions. The larger and more predatory fish tend to accumulate the highest levels and should be avoided particularly by pregnant women and women who are trying to become pregnant. They are; Swordfish, Shark, King Mackerel and Tilefish.

<u>ACTION STEPS FOR THIS CHAPTER</u>

1) Understand the importance of maintaining a stable blood sugar, as nature intended.
2) Realize that there are 2 strategies to maintain a stable blood sugar: 1) Pick the right type of carbohydrates. 2) Always consume some protein, some fat and some carbohydrate at each meal.
3) Pick your proteins from the "Best Choices" and "OK Choices" lists while doing your best to strictly limit protein sources from the "Avoid" list.

Chapter 3:

Fat: The Misunderstood Macronutrient

Fat is without a doubt the most misunderstood nutrient in the field of nutrition. Fats, also known as lipids, are a wide variety of compounds that share one common trait; they do not readily dissolve in water. Triglycerides are the most common form of fat found in food as well as the human body. A triglyceride consists of a glycerol with three fatty acids. Lipids that are solid at room temperature (like butter) are called fats. Lipids that are liquid at room temperature are called oils (such as olive oil). Some of the major functions of fat include;

1) Providing energy for the body.
2) Storing energy for the body.
3) Insulating and protecting vital organs.
4) Transportation of the fat soluble vitamins (A, D, E and K).

Fat has gotten a <u>bad reputation</u>. Early nutrition research showed that certain fats were associated with an increased risk of heart disease and cancer. Another knock against fat is that it is very calorie dense, providing 9 calories per gram as compared to protein and carbohydrate, which provide 4 calories per gram. For these reasons, the main thrust of nutrition advice in the 1980's and 1990's was to drastically reduce the amount of fat in our diets. The motivating force behind this advice was to prevent a variety of diseases and decrease the incidence of obesity.

However, making such blanket recommendations concerning dietary fat was akin to throwing out the baby with the bath water. Let's start with the weight gain issue. It was assumed that the higher intakes of dietary fat were related to obesity. Not necessarily. In this country, the percent of fat in our diet has slowly dropped from 40% to 34% of calories over the past few decades. In this time the rates of obesity have skyrocketed. While there are other important factors at play such as physical activity and total calories, this statistic certainly doesn't support the theory that decreasing the percentage of fat in the diet will have a major effect on weight loss.

A variety of epidemiological studies have shown that there is not a strong association between percent of fat consumed and body weight. In other words, the percentage of fat in your diet has no real influence on your risk of being obese. This is very likely a surprise to most people. I do admit that the amount of fat needs to be monitored in the diet, but in my years of clinical experience and research, I am not at all convinced that a low fat diet is the path to permanent weight loss or greater health.

On to disease risk. I won't argue that certain fats increase the risk of heart disease. What may be surprising is that other fats significantly decrease the risk of heart disease, particularly when substituted for more refined carbohydrates. The association between fat and cancer is also controversial. Recent studies that were more carefully conducted than earlier research have weakened the hypothesis that dietary fat causes cancer.

Let's get this straightened out! There are four types of fat in our diets. Three of these are natural and one is man-made. It is imperative that you get to know these well. Let's start with the man-made fat; partially hydrogenated vegetable oil or trans fat. Trans fat is produced through the commercial hydrogenation of polyunsaturated oils (plant oils). Hydrogen is bubbled through the oil at a certain pressure and in the presence of a nickel catalyst. This changes the chemical structure of the fat. What this means for us is that our body has to deal with an unnatural fat that is incorporated into our cell structures and membranes. A wide variety of negative health effects can occur with high consumption of trans fat. Research has shown that high trans fat intake is associated with increased risk of heart disease, diabetes and possibly some cancers.

Why Are Oils Hydrogenated?

There are a variety of reasons why manufacturers use hydrogenated oils in food products;

1) Hydrogenation removes essential fatty acids such as linoleic and alpha linolenic acid. These fatty acids tend to oxidize over time, which can turn the fat rancid. Therefore, a big reason for the use of hydrogenated oils is to prolong shelf life.
2) Hydrogenation increases the melting point of oil so that the product is solid at 25° Celsius. This acts to improve the texture and consistency of many commercially prepared foods.
3) Using this type of oil is cheaper for the manufacturers.

Where Are Trans Fats Found?

Believe it or not, some trans fats are found in nature. A tiny percent of dairy fat is trans. However, this amount is generally considered too small to produce significant negative health effects. By far the largest contributors to trans fat in the American diet are the commercially prepared oils found in fried and baked food and margarines. Following is a list of some common foods that contain a high percentage of trans fatty acids:

Foods High In Trans Fat
Doughnuts and Pastries
French Fries and Fried Chicken
Potato Chips and Similar Snacks
Imitation Cheese
Margarine
Candy

After a great deal of lobbying by consumer advocate groups, trans fat is now required to appear on food labels. You can find it as a subcategory under "Fats". This is great news. Because trans fats are known to be unhealthy, the requirement of listing it on food labels will influence manufacturers to eliminate it from their products. After all, they don't want their product to be perceived as unhealthy. However, trans fat continues to appear in many food items so if you find it listed, avoid this product as if it will shorten your life because that is exactly what it has the potential to do.

As more is learned about the negative effects of trans fats, a number of the more responsible manufacturers are indeed making attempts to avoid or limit the use of trans fats. McDonald's has recently eliminated trans fat from its food items as has Frito Lay (makers of Doritos, Lay's Chips and Fritos). Taco Bell, Wendy's and Kentucky Fried Chicken have also removed trans fat from their restaurants. Become a label reader and do your best to avoid the dangerous partially hydrogenated vegetable oils.

Saturated Fat

Saturated fats are fats that contain no double bonds. All of the carbons are saturated with hydrogen. They are found, for the most part, in animal products. In general, saturated fats tend to raise LDL cholesterol levels. Research has shown that high levels of saturated fat may increase one's risk of heart disease. Although it is not necessary to completely avoid saturated fat, it is wise to limit intake. Sources of saturated fat include; fatty cuts of steak and other red meat, butter, full fat dairy products like whole milk, ice cream, cheese and whole yogurt. Bacon and fatty cold cuts are also high in saturated fat.

Monounsaturated Fat

Monounsaturated fats have a slightly different structure than other fats. They contain one double bond and therefore not all of their carbons are saturated with hydrogen. You'll find these types of fatty acids in olive oil and canola oil, as well as a variety of nuts and avocados.

Finally, the health effects of monounsaturated fats are being revealed and accepted. I mentioned earlier that a blanket statement to avoid all fats was erroneous. Our first clue as to the health benefits of monounsaturated fats came from cross-sectional ecological studies. These are very simple studies where researchers look at rates of disease among different countries and compare intakes of certain nutrients.

When these studies were carried out, we were expecting to see that the more fat a country consumed, the higher the rates of heart disease and stroke. This held true for some countries, like America, we ate a lot of fat and suffered from a lot of heart disease. However, there were other countries, particularly the Mediterranean regions of Greece and Italy, where comparatively large amounts of fats were consumed yet rates of these diseases were among the lowest in the world.

Take Greece for example. There are parts of Greece where 40-50% of the daily calories come from fat, significantly more than Americans are consuming. We would expect the Greeks to have much more heart disease if fat was a big player in the disease process. They don't. Their rates are much lower than ours. Why this discrepancy? In America, the types of foods we eat are very high in saturated fat and trans fat. In Greece, most of the fat comes from olive oil, a mono-unsaturated fat.

There are people who argue; "It must be genetics. There is something about the Greek people that naturally protects them from heart disease." A gift from mother nature perhaps. Well this turned out to be untrue. Another type of study is called a migrant study. When people leave their native country and emigrate to other cultures, it gives researchers a great opportunity to check the genetic influence on disease. If you keep your low rates of disease after adopting another culture's diet and health habits, then you know that genetics are at play. If your rates of disease climb towards the rates in the new country, then you know it wasn't genes at all, but lifestyle. When Greeks and Italians come to America and adopt our diet, their rates of heart disease increase to our levels. So clearly, their native diet and lifestyle were playing a huge role in protecting them from heart disease.

This type of research paved the way for more complicated metabolic studies on the effects of different fats on things like LDL (bad) cholesterol and HDL (good) cholesterol. It turns out that mono-unsaturated fat, when substituted for saturated fat, lowers LDL cholesterol without changing HDL cholesterol. This helps to reduce the risk of heart disease. When monounsaturated fat is substituted for carbohydrate, LDL levels remain the same but HDL levels increase. This also will help reduce the risk of heart disease. In plain English, eating mono-unsaturated fat will lower your risk of heart disease, not increase it. So, why would you want to lower your intake of it?

Polyunsaturated Fat

A similar story was found to be true concerning polyunsaturated fat. These fats are highly similar to monounsaturated fats but instead of having just one double bond, they have two or more. These fats are found in most nuts and plant oils like corn oil, soybean oil and safflower oil. Polyunsaturated fats, like monounsaturated fats, have been shown to have a beneficial effect on blood lipids and in studies have reduced the incidence of heart disease. Omega 3 fatty acids found in fish, canola oil, soybean oil and walnuts are a very special type of polyunsaturated fat that have been shown to reduce the risk of dangerous arrhythmias and to reduce risk of sudden death due to heart disease.

I hope it is becoming obvious that not all fats are created equal. Some like trans fat and saturated fat, have been found to be harmful to our health. Others like monounsaturated and polyunsaturated fats can be beneficial to our health and there is no reason to avoid them. It makes sense that we would want to limit our intake of saturated and trans fat and increase our intake of the more healthful mono and polyunsaturated fats. Fat also has another great feature. It helps to stabilize your blood sugar by slowing down the rate of stomach emptying. With the addition of fat, carbohydrates consumed will raise blood sugar much more slowly. Remember, just as with protein, you want to be sure to include one source of fat at each and every meal. So here are the best choices and choices to avoid for our all too misunderstood friend fat.

Best Choices

Olive Oil	Pistachios
Canola Oil	Macadamia Nuts
Corn Oil	Any Other Nut
Sunflower Oil	Sunflower Seeds
Safflower Oil	Pumpkin Seeds
Soybean Oil	Avocados
Flaxseed Oil	Peanut Butter
Other Vegetable Oils	Almond Butter
Peanuts	Cashew Butter
Almonds	Olivio
Walnuts	Smart Balance
Cashews	Other Butter
Hazel Nuts	Substitutes

Avoid*

Whole Milk	Snack Chips
Whole Cheese	Pies
Whole Yogurt	Cakes
Whole Cottage Cheese	Cookies
Ice Cream	Crackers
Butter	Chocolate
Margarine	Hamburger
Palm Oil	Steak
Coconut Oil	Salami
French Fries	Bologna
Onion Rings	Pepperoni
Chicken Fingers	Pastrami
Fish Sticks	Any Trans Fat

*These are foods that are known to adversely affect your health due to excessively high levels of saturated and/or trans fat.

<u>ACTION STEPS FOR THIS CHAPTER</u>

1) Don't be scared of fat. If chosen wisely, it can improve your health and facilitate weight loss.
2) Stay away from the unhealthy trans and saturated fats.
3) Choose healthy mono and polyunsaturated fats from the "Best Choice" list at each meal.

Chapter 4

Carbohydrate: The Most Important Macronutrient

The type of carbohydrate that you put into your body can literally make or break your goal of lasting weight loss. Pay very close attention to this chapter! Let's start from the very top. So, what is a carbohydrate? Carbohydrates are composed of carbon, hydrogen and oxygen in the ratio of 1:2:1. Simpler forms of carbohydrates are known as sugars, while more complex forms of carbohydrate are called starches. The main function of carbohydrate is to provide energy for the body and to prevent the breakdown of protein.

The type of carbohydrate that human beings consume has changed dramatically over the years. While we were still evolving, the majority of carbohydrates we ate were fruits and vegetables in their whole form, beans, other legumes and grains that were highly unrefined. As man became more civilized, this all changed; for the worse!

Back before refrigeration and food preservatives, the transport and storage of food was a huge problem. Whole grains contain a small amount of fat that shortens the amount of time it takes for the grain to spoil. By refining the grain, this fat is removed. Therefore, early attempts to refine grains were initiated by the noblest of intentions; to keep food edible longer so fewer people would starve. Thankfully, for most of this country, starvation isn't a huge issue. If anything, there is too much food available.

Biochemistry 101

Let me give you a very brief lesson on what happens to your blood sugar when you eat a carbohydrate. Once you consume a carbohydrate, your blood sugar levels begin to rise. Our body works within a relatively narrow frame of blood sugar. You've got a problem if it goes too high, and you've got a problem if it goes too low. For this reason, the body releases insulin to lower your blood sugar. The amount of insulin released depends on the type and amount of carbohydrate consumed. Some carbohydrates cause the release of large amounts of insulin while others cause a smaller amount of insulin to be released.

When the right type of carbohydrate is consumed, insulin does its job well and lowers blood glucose to normal levels. When the wrong type of carbohydrate is consumed, the large amount of insulin released does its job too well and blood sugar levels drop below that which the body considers normal. When this happens, you'll notice a variety of effects;

1) Your energy drops and you feel tired.
2) Your mood dampens a bit.
3) And most importantly, you get hungry!

The body quickly recognizes that its blood sugar is low. In order to raise it back up, it makes you hungry! The very thing you'll crave is a quick release carbohydrate and the cycle begins again. As mentioned earlier, high insulin levels also promote fat storage. This combination of increased hunger and increased fat storage is devastating to those trying to lose weight.

In summary, all carbohydrates are not created equal! Some will raise your blood sugar really high, really fast, causing the release of large amounts of insulin. Other carbohydrates have a more slow and gradual effect on your blood sugar and do not necessitate a large release of insulin. Enter the glycemic index.

The glycemic index was proposed by Dr. David Jenkins at the University of Toronto in 1981 as a way of classifying carbohydrates. Very simply, it gives a score as to how quickly and how severely a carbohydrate will raise your blood sugar. It all starts by feeding a group of subjects 50 grams of glucose (which is pure sugar) and measuring their blood sugar response. This is the baseline or reference measure. Next, the researchers feed the same people 50 grams of another type of carbohydrate, say a baked potato, and measure their blood sugar response once again.

The glycemic index number is the blood sugar response of that particular carbohydrate relative to the pure glucose reading. For example, the glycemic index of a white baked potato is 78. What that really means is when you eat equal amounts of a white baked potato and pure glucose, the potato results in 78% of the blood sugar response of the pure glucose. This test is repeated for all types of carbohydrate containing foods.

Take a look at this example. Notice how the higher glycemic carbohydrate causes dramatic increases in insulin and glucose levels compared to the lower glycemic carbohydrate.

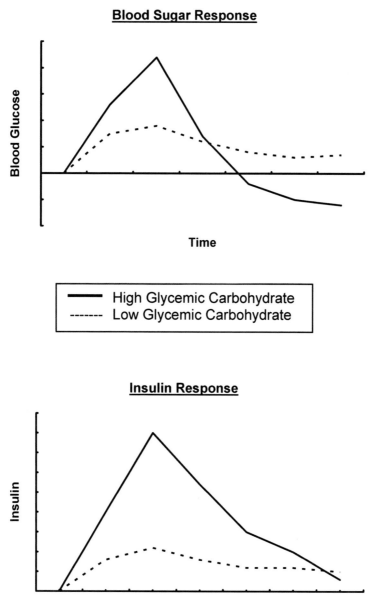

We can use the glycemic index and a related concept called the glycemic load to help us pick our carbohydrates. The glycemic load was proposed by some of my colleagues at Harvard University to shed more light on the concept of high glycemic carbohydrates. The glycemic load is the glycemic index multiplied by the amount of carbohydrate supplied in a typical serving of the food. Therefore, the glycemic load takes into account both the quality and quantity of carbohydrate.

Why is this important? Well, for starters, the glycemic load gives you a more practical look at how a carbohydrate will affect your blood sugar. Most of the foods that have a high glycemic index also have a high glycemic load. For example, white rice has a glycemic index of 91 (which is considered very high) and a glycemic load of 24.8 (also considered very high). White bread has a glycemic index of 70 and a glycemic load of 21, both considered high. On the other end of the spectrum, lentil beans have a low glycemic index of 29 and also a low glycemic load of 5.7 and apples similarly have both a low glycemic index (36) and a low glycemic load (8.1).

However, there are some interesting exceptions. Carrots have a high glycemic index at 71 but the glycemic load of carrots is small at 3.8. This is because carrots have a lot of fiber and water and supply only a small amount of carbohydrate per serving. Hence the lower glycemic load. Remember glycemic load is the product of both the glycemic index and the amount of carbohydrate.

So you can see that some foods with a high glycemic index really won't hurt your blood sugar (because only small amounts of carbohydrate are delivered) while some foods with more moderate glycemic indices (like pasta) will really hurt your blood sugar because of the large amount of carbohydrates delivered in a serving. To aid in the weight loss process, you want to focus on foods with a low glycemic load.

It should not come as a huge surprise that the overwhelming majority of foods with a high glycemic load are man made, refined carbohydrates. The big offenders are bread, pasta, white rice and sugar. Most fruits and vegetables have a much lower glycemic load and will have a milder effect on your blood sugar. This makes sense because fruits, vegetables and legumes are the carbohydrates that were put on the Earth for us to consume. These foods are what we evolved with and it is not surprising that our bodies function best when consuming them.

Therefore, when choosing carbohydrates, we want to focus on lower glycemic load carbohydrates like fruits, vegetables, legumes and whole grains such as brown rice and oatmeal. There are just a few small exceptions. For fruits, any are permitted with the exception of bananas and grapes. They have less fiber than other fruits and are therefore higher glycemic. Certainly don't eliminate them from your diet, just go easy on them. For vegetables, the only notable exception is white potatoes. They are really high glycemic and should be consumed with moderation. Remember Rule #1; Combine your carbohydrate with fat and protein at every meal and snack.

Determinants Of A Foods Glycemic Index

Increases GI	Decreases GI
Processing/Refining food	Addition of fat
Longer cooking times	Addition of protein
	Addition of fiber

As a side note, consuming a diet with a high glycemic load has been shown to increase your risk of type 2 diabetes, coronary heart disease, cancer and even Alzheimer's disease. So, consuming a low glycemic load diet not only will stabilize your blood sugar and insulin levels, it will also help protect you from chronic disease in the future.

Best Choices

Apples	Green Pepper
Oranges	Red Pepper
Pineapple	Olives
Blueberries	Carrots
Strawberries	Spinach
Raspberries	Lettuce
Melon	Peas
Grapefruit	Lentils
Watermelon	Black Beans
Mango	Pink Beans
Papaya	Chick Peas
Kiwi	Hummus
Sweet Potato	Other Beans
Broccoli	Other Fruits
Cauliflower	Other Vegetables
Tomatoes	Brown Rice
Onion	Oatmeal (Not
Radishes	Instant)

OK Choices

Corn

Avoid

White Bread	Other Fruit Juice
Wheat Bread	Soda
Tortillas	Cakes
Wraps	Cookies
Pita Bread	Pies
Pasta	Candy
White Rice	Donuts
Bananas	Ketchup
Grapes	BBQ Sauce
White Potatoes	Steak Sauce
Crackers	Jams
Rice Cakes	Jellies
Popcorn	Sweetened Yogurt
Bagels	Raisins
Pretzels	Other Dried Fruit
Potato Chips	Low Fat Salad
Sugar	Dressing
Orange Juice	Anything Else
Tomato Juice	With Sugar!!!

Right about now you may be saying "I'll never be able to give up bread and sugar! I crave them way too much!" Many people feel this way at the beginning of the program and I will admit that at first it is a challenge to give up these foods. However, it is important to know that when your blood sugar becomes more stable, (usually in just a few weeks) these cravings will go away entirely. I haven't had sugar in over 10 years now and believe me when I tell you I don't even think twice about it anymore, and I had the biggest sweet tooth on Long Island when I was a kid.

In my personal experience and that of my clients, cravings for these refined carbohydrate foods are not psychological but physiological. When you are in "bad blood sugar" you often crave quick release carbohydrates to counter the dip in blood glucose caused by higher levels of insulin. It truly is a vicious cycle. When you are in a state of "good blood sugar" these craving disappear. It is not a question of mental strength or mental weakness. Stabilize your blood sugar and the cravings go away.

Many people are actually addicted to sugar and refined carbohydrates and go through a withdrawal period when giving them up. In the first few weeks of eliminating sugar and refined carbohydrates from your diet you may notice that you are a little more tired and irritable and may even get a headache or two. You'll also have some serious cravings for the foods you are limiting. These symptoms are not serious and will go away on their own after 2 to 3 weeks on the program.

After a few weeks of eating this way, you can once again listen to your hunger to tell you what your body needs. You will no longer get hungry in order to fix your blood sugar. Although it is a bit rough at first, one of the biggest surprises for my clients is that they no longer crave bread, pasta, rice and sugar after just a few weeks. You'll get there too! You just need to tough it out for the first 14 days or so.

Hidden Sugars

Sugar is everywhere! To avoid it, you must become a big time label reader. For example; ketchup, barbeque sauce, steak sauce and low-fat salad dressings are loaded with sugar and need to be avoided. Thankfully, today's food labels are much easier to read than in years past. On the next page is an example of a typical food label. Look under the "carbohydrate" category and you'll see a listing for "sugars". This is the number of grams of sugar in a serving. You want this number to be as close to 0 as possible. Divide this number by 4 and that is the number of teaspoons of sugar found in a serving of that food. In our example there are 18 grams of sugar per serving (4 ½ teaspoons). Stay away from this food for sure!

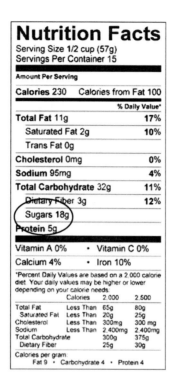

Note that dairy products like milk, plain yogurt and cottage cheese will have a high number under the "sugars" column yet don't taste sweet or have any added sugars. This is because lactose is a naturally occurring sugar found in dairy that does not have an adverse effect on blood glucose, it is low glycemic. So, with dairy you need to look at the list of ingredients and make sure that no other sugars are added in to the product.

Food manufacturers use lots of different names for sugars. Following is a list of ingredients that basically can be translated to **SUGAR**. This is important when reading food labels, rarely will you see the word "sugar" listed as an ingredient.

Sucrose
Molasses
Concentrated Fruit Juice
Corn Syrup
Corn Sweetener
Brown Sugar
Raw Sugar
Cane Syrup
High Fructose Corn Syrup
Dextrose
Fructose
Levulose
Maple Sugar
Turbinado
Honey
Dextrin
Glucose
Galactose
Maltose
Beet Sugar
Cane Sugar

So, there you have it. Carbohydrate quality and quantity are pivotal for those attempting to lose weight. In my opinion, the combination of high glycemic load carbohydrates and low fat diets have much to do with the explosion of obesity in recent years. Decreases in physical activity also play a huge role. But we'll get to that a little bit later!

ACTION STEPS FOR THIS CHAPTER

1) As always, combine a source of fat, protein and carbohydrate at every meal.
2) Focus on low glycemic load carbohydrates from the "Best Choices" list.
3) Become a label reader.
4) Beware of hidden sources of sugars in the foods you eat.
5) Become familiar with all of the words manufacturers use for sugar.

Chapter 5

Putting It All Together:
How To Stabilize Your Blood Sugar

Ok, so now we have an idea of what type of foods we should be eating and what type of foods we should be avoiding in order to lose weight and improve our health. Now let's put it all together. The most important thing to remember is the following;

Consume One Carbohydrate Food, One Fat Food And One Protein Food At Each Meal Or Snack

Why is this so very important? There are several reasons;

1) I want to emphasize enough healthy fat in my client's diet and this is a good way to ensure this will happen.

2) I want to emphasize adequate amounts of lean protein in my client's diet and this is a good way to ensure this will happen.

3) Most Importantly, I want to stabilize blood sugar, which will facilitate weight loss by decreasing cravings and possibly by increasing access to fat stores. The addition of fat and

protein to a carbohydrate food slows the absorption of the carbohydrate into the blood stream and this greatly decreases the swings in blood sugar and insulin levels so common in the American diet. This will also tend to have a nice effect on energy levels and mood.

This is really easy to accomplish. Let's look at all of the macronutrients at once, focusing on the Best and OK choices for each.

Protein Best Choices

Chicken w/o skin	Monkfish
Turkey w/o skin	Flounder
Lean Ham	Other Fish
Pork	Egg Whites
Lobster	Black Beans
Crab	Pink Beans
Scallops	Navy Beans
Clams	Chick Peas
Mussels	Lentils
Salmon	Other Beans
Scrod	Soy Protein
Chilean Sea Bass	

Protein OK Choices

Skim Milk	Filet Mignon
Low-fat Cottage Cheese	Lean Ground Beef
Low-fat Cheese	Lean Roast Beef
Low-fat Plain Yogurt	Shrimp
Whole Eggs	Tuna

Fat Best Choices

Olive Oil	Pistachios
Canola Oil	Macadamia Nuts
Corn Oil	Any Other Nut
Sunflower Oil	Sunflower Seeds
Safflower Oil	Pumpkin Seeds
Soybean Oil	Avocados
Flaxseed Oil	Peanut Butter
Other Vegetable Oils	Almond Butter
Peanuts	Cashew Butter
Almonds	Olivio
Walnuts	Smart Balance
Cashews	Other Butter
Hazel Nuts	Substitutes

Carbohydrate Best Choices

Apples	Green Pepper
Oranges	Red Pepper
Pineapple	Olives
Blueberries	Carrots
Strawberries	Spinach
Raspberries	Lettuce
Melon	Peas
Grapefruit	Lentils
Watermelon	Black Beans
Mango	Pink Beans
Papaya	Chick Peas
Kiwi	Hummus
Sweet Potato	Other Beans
Broccoli	Other Fruits
Cauliflower	Other Vegetables
Tomatoes	Brown Rice
Onion	Oatmeal (Not
Radishes	Instant)

Carbohydrate OK Choices

Corn

When planning a meal, pick one food from each list. Try to vary them on a day to day basis but definitely let your tastes guide you. Let's say this is day one of your new life. You want to start the dietary changes today and, logically, breakfast is your first meal of your first day. First, pick a breakfast protein from the list of acceptable protein foods; say low fat cottage cheese. Now move over to the fat category and select whatever you want, some peanuts for example. Lastly look at the carbohydrate group and pick a food-an apple will do nicely. We will worry about portions in just a minute. For now, understand the choice of a food from each category as being a critical part of the dietary regimen.

Breakfast
Protein---Low fat cottage cheese
Fat---Peanuts
Carbohydrate---Apple

Lunch
Protein--Grilled chicken
Fat--Olive oil
Carbohydrate--Salad vegetables (lettuce, tomatoes, etc)

Dinner
Protein--Salmon
Fat--Canola oil
Carbohydrate--Brown rice and broccoli

Now let's move to lunch. An ideal lunch would be the following; a big salad with lots of vegetables (carbohydrate), some grilled chicken on top (protein) and some olive oil and vinegar dressing (fat). Get the idea? One from each category, any one you want. How about dinner? Let's start with a nice piece of salmon (protein), a sweet potato and broccoli sautéed in canola oil (carbohydrate and fat). That is how it works. Pretty easy, right? It will take a little getting used to but once you get going, you'll find it is a flexible way to eat filled with a variety of delicious, healthy foods.

I suggest keeping a copy of the Best Choices, OK Choices and Those To Avoid on your refrigerator. This will help you to keep your focus on proper food selection, particularly when you are planning your shopping. Following are a few more sample days on the plan.

Day 2 Breakfast	Day 3 Breakfast	Day 4 Breakfast	Day 5 Breakfast
Protein- Eggs (omelet)	Protein-Plain low fat yogurt	Protein-1% or skim milk	Protein-Turkey bacon
Carbohydrate-Mixed Vegetables	Carbohydrate-Mixed berries	Carbohydrate-Oatmeal	Carbohydrate-Pear
Fat-Egg yolks are your fat	Fat- Chopped walnuts	Fat-Peanut butter	Fat-Sunflower seeds
Lunch	**Lunch**	**Lunch**	**Lunch**
Protein- Tuna fish	Protein-Lentils (lentil soup)	Protein- Chili (lean ground beef or turkey)	Protein-Fish (brown rice sushi)
Carbohydrate-Cut vegetables	Carbohydrate-Lentils	Carbohydrate-Vegetables in chili	Carbohydrate-Brown Rice
Fat-Mayonnaise	Fat-Vegetable oil in soup	Fat-Vegetable oil in chili	Fat- Avocado
Dinner	**Dinner**	**Dinner**	**Dinner**
Protein-Chicken Breast	Protein-Turkey burger-no roll	Protein-Shrimp stir fry	Protein-Filet mignon
Carbohydrate-Broccoli, side salad	Carbohydrate-Tomato, onion mushrooms	Carbohydrate-Vegetables, brown rice	Carbohydrate-Sweet potato, string beans
Fat-Olive oil	Fat-Guacamole	Fat- Canola oil	Fat- Olive oil (to sauté string beans)

Portions

I never have my clients weigh their food or get too crazy about portion sizes, but a few guidelines are really important. Let's look at each of the macro-nutrients and talk a bit about portion sizes.

Protein

While at Harvard, a fair amount of my research was focused on low carbohydrate diets like Atkins. On a low carb diet, protein is allowed in unlimited quantities and you are encouraged to eat as much as you want. In randomized trials studying people consuming a low carb diet, I found it interesting that protein intake never really exceeded 20-25% of calories. These people were allowed to eat as much protein as they wanted to and yet they really didn't go overboard. I have noticed the same thing with my clients.

The reason for this ends up being quite simple. Protein contains nitrogen, which is difficult for the human body to process and can be quite toxic at high levels. For this reason the body tends to limit the protein that it will have to process. In other words, you won't overeat protein. So the take home message here regarding protein portions is to eat protein until you are full. Your body won't let you go higher than 20-25% of calories, which is just where I want you to be.

Carbohydrates

The vast majority of carbohydrates on this plan are very low in calories. Fruits and vegetables contain a lot of fiber and water. For this reason, there really are no limits to the amounts of fruits, vegetables and other allowable carbs on this program. Eat until you are full. A bowl of broccoli will run you about 130 calories while the same size bowl of pasta can be 600 calories. Load up on a wide variety of fruits and vegetables without stressing too much about portions.

Fats

Fat is the only one of the three macronutrients that I recommend very strict portion guidelines. Having too little fat in your diet will cause you to have blood sugar issues. Having too much fat in your diet will cause you to have calorie issues. Follow these portions to avoid both scenarios.

<u>For Women</u>
1) If you are having oil on your salad or to sauté your vegetables; 1 tablespoon will do it.
2) If you are having nuts; 7 large nuts (cashews, macadamia nuts, walnuts, almonds) will do; 14 small nuts like peanuts or pistachio nuts will do.
3) If you are having nut butter, 1 heaping tea-spoon.

    4) If you are having avocado as your fat source, ¼ if it's a large avocado and ½ if it's a small avocado.

<u>For Men</u>
    1) If you are having oil on your salad or to sauté your vegetables, 1½ tablespoons will do it.
    2) Nuts: 12 large and 24 small.
    3) Nut butter: 2 heaping teaspoons.
    4) Avocado: ½ if it's a large avocado and ¾ if it's a small avocado.

A Note Concerning Beans And Eggs

Most foods fit neatly into either the protein, fat or carbohydrate category. A few foods overlap and really fit into 2 groups. Eggs, eaten whole with the yolk, provide both protein and fat. Therefore, if you have eggs at a meal, they will satisfy both your protein and fat requirement and all you'll need is a carb. If you are just using the egg whites, then count them just as your protein. Beans and other legumes similarly are a good source of both protein and carbohydrate and should be counted as a source in both groups when planning meals.

Good Foods To Always Keep On Hand

As you can see, this program allows a lot of freedom to choose foods you enjoy, foods that taste great and have the benefits of not only helping you lose weight but increasing your energy and health in general. It is important to think about your meals well ahead of time and when you shop, make sure you have all the tools you need to construct your meal plan for the day. It's always a good idea to keep the following items well stocked in order to stay on track.

Proteins- sliced turkey breast or other low fat deli meats like ham, etc. Tuna, eggs, chicken, low fat dairy such as plain non-fat yogurt, skim milk and low fat cottage cheese.

Fats- olive oil, canola oil, peanut butter, nuts, seeds.

Carbohydrates- a wide variety of fruits and vegetables, beans, old fashioned slow cooked oatmeal, brown rice.

If you need a quick meal, grab a few slices of turkey breast, a handful of nuts and an apple and you're out the door. If you need a quick breakfast when running late for work, have a few spoonfuls of low fat cottage cheese or plain yogurt, grab some sunflower seeds and a pear and you're on your way.

The key is to keep on hand the raw materials to build your meals. We all run into trouble when we have nothing in the house and stop for something on the way to work. What you grab for convenience is almost never as good as what you'd have if you took a little time to plan your meals.

So this concludes the all important diet component of the plan. Now it is time to focus on the next 2 areas; cardiovascular training and resistance training.

<u>ACTION STEPS FOR THIS CHAPTER</u>

1) Combine a fat, a protein and a carbohydrate at each meal or snack.

2) When it comes to protein and carbohydrate, don't worry much about portions. Eat until you are full. Once your blood sugar stabilizes, your hunger will reflect what your body needs.

3) Strictly follow the fat portions. Too little fat and you'll have blood sugar issues, too much fat and you'll have calorie issues.

4) Remember that eggs with the yolks will count as both your fat and your protein and beans count as both your protein and carbohydrate.

Chapter 6

Cardiovascular Exercise:
Burn Those Calories

After your diet, cardio is the 2nd most important factor that will determine your success in losing weight and keeping it off. First of all, cardiovascular training burns calories. This will help to access the undesirable fat stores you are looking to reduce. Believe it or not, this isn't even the major benefit of cardiovascular exercise. For about 12 hours after a cardio session you burn more calories than you would if you had not exercised. This happens for a variety of reasons including the reloading of energy substrate and the repair of micro damage to utilized muscle groups. This metabolic boost, in my opinion, is the real benefit to cardiovascular training.

There are 3 basic components to a cardiovascular exercise program that need to be addressed; 1) Type 2) Frequency/Duration 3) Intensity.

Note

Before we get started, I would recommend that you mention to your doctor that you are starting an exercise program and want to make sure you are medically cleared to do so. I don't say this to cover my butt but to cover yours. This is very important and often I will not recommend any exercise for a new client until I receive medical clearance. I will be asking you to work at a moderate to high intensity with regards to heart rate and it's important that you have the confidence that it is safe to do so. Now let's break down the 3 parts of the cardio program.

Type

The type of cardiovascular exercise you engage in is entirely up to you. Let your individual preferences guide you. However, do realize that some exercises are more effective in helping you to achieve your goal of lasting weight loss.

Best Choices
Walking or Walk/Jog Intervals
Elliptical Trainer
Stair Climber

Secondary Choices
Bike
Roller Blading
Ice Skating

Secondary Choices- continued
Swimming
Jogging
Aerobic Dance

You can see the types of cardio are broken down into Best Choices and Secondary Choices. As the name implies, the Best Choice exercises will be your main source of cardio, the one you'll do the most consistently. These exercises are typically easy to learn, are not weight supported and therefore force you to work harder and expend more calories. These choices also provide minimal impact on your joints.

Walking or Walking/Jogging Intervals

If you are 20-30 pounds overweight and/or a little bit older (older than 50) you may want to start with walking as your source of cardio. It is easy (we all know how to do it), convenient (weather permitting-you can just head outside) and cheap (a good pair of running or walking sneakers is all you will need). All in all, walking is a great way to get started. After a while, however, walking will no longer be intense enough for you to continue losing weight. At this time you may want to graduate to a walk/jog interval training program. With this type of program, you walk for 3 minutes and then jog for 2 minutes and repeat throughout the cardio session. You get the benefit of burning more calories than walking without the continual high impact of running.

Once you hit the point where walking is no longer intense enough (you'll know it's time when the scale stops moving downward), you can continue to utilize walking as your main cardio choice but you'll have to greatly increase your time commitment. At this point, I'll give my clients one minute toward their cardio goal for every 2 they walk. So, if your goal for cardio is 200 minutes a week, you will need to walk 400 minutes.

Elliptical Trainer

You may have seen these machines on television or at the gym. God bless the man or woman who invented the elliptical trainer! It truly gives you the best of both worlds. You get the calorie burning potential of a more strenuous method of cardio (like jogging) with very low impact. There is minimal stress on joints with these machines. The movement is very fluid, and a lot of fun. I feel like I'm working as hard as I do when I run but feel none of the impact. This is usually my first choice of cardio if my clients can get access to one. Just about every gym has these machines and there are now lower costing models for the home (The Tony Little Gazelle Edge is under $100). Give this one a try!!

Stair Climber

The stair climber is also a great form of cardio that qualifies for the Best Choice group. These have been around for years and do a good job of burning calories while keeping the impact on your joints to a minimum.

Secondary Forms Of Cardio

The secondary forms of cardio are adequate choices yet are not quite what we are looking for as far as a consistent choice of cardiovascular exercise. Many of these exercises either require a lot of skill, have an increased risk of injury, are expensive or inconvenient for one reason or another. These modes of cardio are fine for a substitute now and again (once or twice a week) but I wouldn't recommend them to be done on a consistent basis.

Bike Riding

There are 2 types of bike riding. Riding outdoors on the street can be dangerous and is highly dependent on the weather. Riding indoor on a stationary bike is safe and independent of the weather, but in both cases, the bike is supporting your weight so you burn far fewer calories than you would with a primary form of exercise. Now and again this is OK but certainly not as your major source of cardio. If you absolutely love to bike or spin, you can count 1 minute toward your cardio goal for every 2 minutes you bike or spin.

Rollerblading

This is a great, lower impact form of cardio that burns tons of calories and is loads of fun (I'm a hockey player and love skating in all of its forms). The reason why it is not on the primary list is that it takes a fair amount of skill, carries with it a significant risk of injury and is highly dependent on the weather. Ditto for ice skating.

Swimming

Swimming is also a great form of cardio. You work every muscle in your body. It's on the secondary list largely because of accessibility issues. Not many people can get to a pool multiple times a week. Furthermore, since the water is supporting your weight, you're not burning as many calories as you would with an upright form of exercise like elliptical training.

Jogging

Jogging is a little more advanced and I normally do not recommend it to my clients as a long term choice. When we run, we can put up to 6 times our body weight on our joints. I weigh 185 pounds so when I run, I am putting the equivalent of 1100 pounds on my joints. I don't think that we were designed to do this for long periods of time. Just about every client that I've had that insists on running for their major source of cardio, and I'm talking for years here, sustains an overuse injury that keeps them on the sideline at some point and usually repeatedly. It's a shame too, because you burn a lot of calories when you run.

If they really want to run, I advise my clients to engage in an interval type training. I have them walk for 3 minutes and then jog for 2 minutes and repeat. This gives you the best of both worlds; you get an increased calorie burn from the jogging without the chronic stress on the joints.

Aerobic Dance

Aerobic classes can be an effective source of cardio but there are usually a few problems with them. Often, they are high impact and tough on the joints. Furthermore, these classes are usually stop and go with regards to heart rate and I'm generally looking for a more consistent heart rate demand. If your aerobics class is easy on the joints and you truly are working hard the whole time, then this can be your main source of cardio. If not, limit yourself to one or two classes a week and pick a primary source of cardio.

Frequency And Duration

There are a lot of opinions concerning the frequency and duration of the cardio session. Some trainers feel that you should work out every day, others say that you should work out in the morning and still others suggest splitting the workout into several smaller sessions throughout the day. While there are merits to each of these theories, I have found that in practice the only really important factor is total minutes of cardio per week. I give my clients a certain number of minutes that need to get done and it is entirely up to them how they do it. I care about the intensity and the total minutes, that's all.

A common number of cardio minutes that I'd give to a male weight loss client is 150 minutes a week. I don't care if he does 6 times a week for 25 minutes, 4 times a week for 38 minutes or 3 times a week for 50 minutes. The truth of the matter is that it doesn't affect the results too much either way. However he can fit it into his life is fine by me. I care only that the minutes get done consistently.

The number of cardio minutes you will need to lose weight is highly subjective and will change as you progress toward a more healthy weight. If you have a lot of weight to lose, many pounds will come off with lower levels of cardio. Eventually, more cardio will become necessary to keep the scale moving in the right direction. Having said that, here is a general re-commendation;

Women

I must say that when it comes to weight loss, I do feel a little bit sorry for the ladies. Because men have more muscle than women, they have a much easier time losing weight and can get away with far lower levels of cardio. But you know what they say: "That which we obtain too easily, we esteem too lightly". In my experience, most women will lose the vast majority of their weight getting 250 minutes of cardio a week. That is 36 minutes a day, 7 days a week or 42 minutes a day, 6 days a week or 50 minutes a day, 5 days a week. I know that this sounds like a lot, and it is, but believe me it is necessary.

How do we know this amount is necessary? We need look no further than the National Weight Control Registry. The NWCR is an ongoing study established in 1994 by collaborators from Brown Medical School and the University of Colorado. This study is the largest prospective investigation of long term successful weight loss and weight maintenance. Participants have lost at least 30 pounds and kept the weight off for a minimum of 1 year. Over 5000 subjects are being tracked and the average weight loss is 66 pounds kept off for 6 years. This is pretty impressive weight loss and more importantly, maintenance of the loss. The researchers periodically publish results describing how these people have maintained their weight loss. Well guess what, over 90% of them exercise an hour or more per day. I have observed the same with my clients over the last decade or so. The bottom line is this: Those who lose weight and keep it off do a lot of cardio! We all need to accept this fact.

Don't jump right into this amount. Work your way up to it. If you are really out of shape or deconditioned, start with 120 minutes the first week then progress to 175 minutes in week 2 and then hit the 250 by week 3.

If you hit a plateau that lasts 2 weeks or longer and your diet has been good and you've done your resistance training religiously and you've followed the lifestyle guidelines, you may want to increase your cardio by 10-20 minutes a week to get the scale moving again. Again, in most cases, 250 minutes is all you'll need. The maximum cardio you should do is 300-350 minutes per week. If you do more than this, you run the risk of breaking down muscle tissue for energy which will hurt you in the long run by decreasing your metabolism. If you hit this maximum level and your weight is still not where you want it to be, cardio is not the problem. Look into your diet, lifestyle habits or resistance program and chances are one of these facets of the program are slowing you down.

Men

Men get off easy when it comes to cardio. Usually 150 minutes is all that will be needed to satisfy the cardiovascular component of their program. As with the ladies, if you are out of shape or deconditioned, go easy at first. Start with 75 minutes the first week then progress to 120 minutes the second week and then progress to the full 150 by the third week.

If you hit a plateau that lasts 2 weeks or longer and your diet has been good and you've done your resistance training religiously and you've followed the lifestyle guidelines, you may want to increase your cardio by 10-20 minutes a week to get the scale moving again. Again, in most cases, 150 minutes is all you'll need.

Intensity

The intensity of your cardiovascular program is probably the most important component of the three elements. If you are not working at the proper level of intensity for you, the weight loss process will be much less efficient. Generally, you want to work just below your anaerobic lactate threshold, which is between 70-85% of your maximum heart rate. You may have heard of people taking their heart rate or calculating their target heart rate zone to gauge intensity. Well, I'm not going to ask you to do that. #1) It is complicated. #2) The maximum heart rate formula does not apply to a large segment of the population. #3) There are easier ways.

So how will we measure your intensity? There are a few simple ways to clue you in to whether or not you are working as hard as you need to be.

1) <u>Are you sweating?</u> After about 5 minutes into your workout, you should be starting to sweat. If you are not, then you have to pick up the pace. You don't need to be dripping sweat to satisfy this test, but you should notice some sweat at least under your armpits. Not the most pleasant test, but it works.

2) <u>Can you talk?</u> Another simple way to gauge intensity is the talk test. In the middle of your workout, try talking to someone (or yourself if

need be). If you are taking a breath after every 2 words, you're working too hard and need to slow down. If you are able to string multiple sentences together without stopping for air, you need to pick it up. You should be able to say a normal length sentence without taking a breath. But you should need to take a breath after this sentence.

3) <u>Ratings of perceived exertion.</u> When you are working out, stop and ask yourself: "How hard am I working on a scale from 1 to 10? " On the following page you can see a sample rating of perceived exertion scale with descriptions for each level. The level of 7 and 8 corresponds with both the sweating and the talk test. Shoot for that.

Level 10---All out maximal sprint. You could last at this level for maybe 30 seconds.

Level 9---Close to maximal effort. You could last a few minutes at this pace.

Level 8--- Sweat test/talk test

Level 7--- Sweat test/talk test

Level 6---Walking very fast. As if you're late for an appointment.

Level 5---Walking moderately fast

Level 4---Walking normally

Level 3---Walking at a slow pace

Level 2---Standing still

Level 1---Sitting down and reading

Level 0---Sleeping ☺

The key to all of this is to pay attention to your intensity. Get the most out of your cardio session by working at the proper level.

Additional Benefits Of Cardio

Imagine if a new medication was introduced to the market that helped you lose weight. Imagine if this medicine also decreased the risk of heart disease, stroke, diabetes, Alzheimer's disease and cancer.

Imagine if it would also reduce blood pressure, improve blood cholesterol profiles, increase your energy and reduce both anxiety and depression. This drug would also combat insomnia, improve your sex drive and actually increase your confidence and self esteem. Sounds like a dream right? Too good to be true?

This last paragraph pretty much sums up the many benefits of cardiovascular exercise. If a drug like this actually came to market, I bet in 2 months 90% of the adult US population would have a prescription for it. Amazingly, a recent study showed that more than half of Americans don't attain the recommended levels of physical activity to provide these health benefits. And 1 in 4 reported absolutely no leisure time physical activity. What a shame.

Tips For Getting Your Cardio Done

I've been working with clients who want to lose weight for well over 10 years. I know that it is not easy to fit the required amount of cardio into your busy life. I must say that those who consistently found a way to get their cardio done were much more likely to succeed than those who kept finding excuses as to why they couldn't fit it into their busy lives.

In general, the most cardio I ever have a client do is 45 minutes 5 to 6 times a week. Trust me, I know this is a time commitment but you must work on making it a priority. Getting this cardio done consistently will improve just about every area of your life; your health, your energy, your mood, even your self esteem. You get a lot back from this investment. And remember this is the most you'll have to do. Once you hit your goal weight, you'll be able to reduce your cardio minutes by about 30%. So here are some tips to help you get cardio into your life on a consistent basis.

#1) <u>Make it a priority.</u> First of all, consciously understand the importance of getting your cardio done for your health and weight loss goals.

#2) <u>Keep a record of your daily cardio minutes.</u> Write your minutes of cardio in a journal, add them up each week and see how well you did. There is something about seeing things in black and white that helps us to be more accountable. This can also be a tool to adjust your program. Look for patterns. Maybe you'll see that Monday is so busy that you keep missing your cardio; make sure that is one of your days off.

It's important to have the right frame of mind when keeping cardio logs. Don't expect them to be perfect. Don't beat yourself up if your log is not exactly as it should be. We all slip up with our diet and exercise, that's human nature (even I do!). See the log for what it is; a valuable tool to help you track your highs and lows and your overall progress. Don't feel like you're being graded here.

#3) <u>Consider getting a piece of cardiovascular equipment for your home.</u> If financially possible, I always advise my clients to get some type of cardio equipment in their home. There are several reasons for this. If you are doing cardio 5 or 6 times a week during your initial weight loss phase, it can be difficult if not impossible to get to the gym all of those days. If you have a piece of equipment at home, you can hop on for 15 minutes here and 20 minutes there and get the job done. It also takes the weather out of the equation if you are currently exercising outdoors.

There is no need to get a very expensive machine. There are a number of home models ranging in price from $100-$200. I currently recommend the Tony Little Gazelle Edge to my clients. This is an in-home elliptical trainer that costs under $100. I have one myself and love it.

Consider it an investment in your health and your future. If you took one year's worth of gym dues, you'd be surprised at how nicely you can make a little gym in your home. A nice piece of cardio equipment, a simple flat bench and some dumbbells will cost less than many gym's yearly dues and last a lifetime, or close to it. Remember we need consistency above all else. Make it easy for yourself by working out at home if at all possible.

#4) <u>Killing 2 birds with 1 stone.</u> Try to combine your cardio with something you already do everyday. Let me tell you a little story. Several years back I had a client named Beverly who was trying to lose weight. Beverly had the diet down very well and I was working with her twice a week in her home lifting weights so her resistance training program was dead on. She was a very, very busy women working as a school teacher and had many family obligations. She just couldn't get her cardio in and this fact was greatly slowing down her results.

I let her know that her inability to get the requisite cardio was slowing her progress. She said she really wanted to get it done, but she just couldn't seem to fit it in. I asked her about her daily schedule. After work got out she'd rush home to start preparing dinner or baby sit her grandson or one of a million other things. She also mentioned that she always watched her favorite TV show, "Who wants to be a millionaire", with her husband. Bingo- I said to her "Hey Beverly, why don't you put a TV in front of your treadmill and get your cardio done as you watch the show?". Well that was the trick. Beverly never missed that show and after this small adjustment, she never missed her cardio either. She quickly hit her goal weight and when I left her, she was on a nice maintenance program.

Look at your daily schedule. Is there something that you do every day for 30 or 40 minutes that you could combine with your cardio? Is there a TV show that you watch, maybe the news? You can easily read on most pieces of cardio today, why not combine your daily look at the newspaper with your cardio. I've been known to return phone calls and even study while doing cardio when my schedule becomes particularly busy. Having a piece of cardio equipment in your home makes it surprisingly easy to hit your goal for the week.

The bottom line is that if you make your cardio a priority, you can find a way to fit it in. "I'm too busy" is not a good excuse. Ironically, it is usually my most busy clients that find ways to get their cardio done because it becomes a priority to them when they realize they must do it to reach their goals. Make it a priority for you too!!!!!

ACTION STEPS FOR THIS CHAPTER

1) Talk to your doctor and get clearance before starting any exercise program.
2) Pick a "Primary" source of cardio for most of your work. These choices give you more bang for your weight loss buck.
3) Get your minutes in each week. Generally 250 for women and 150 for men.
4) Work at the proper intensity. Remember "The Talk Test", "The Sweat Test" and "The Ratings Of Perceived Exertion".
5) Keep a record of your cardio minutes and add them up each week to stay on course.
6) Consider an inexpensive piece of cardio equipment for your home and try to combine it with something you already do such as TV watching, returning phone calls, etc.

Chapter 7

Resistance Training:
Build And Tone Muscle

Resistance training or weight training is the last but certainly not least component of your weight loss program. More often than not it is completely ignored by those trying to lose weight. A lot of myths and misconceptions are part of the reason why this is so. Let's start from the beginning; Why is resistance training so vital to the weight loss effort?

As you may know, the body can broadly be broken down into 2 components; fat mass and lean body mass. Fat mass is rather self-explanatory; it's your body fat. Lean body mass is basically everything else; your bones, muscles, organs, connective tissue, etc. There are lots of differences between the functions of fat and lean body mass. That is not really within the scope of this chapter. What you need to know is that lean body mass burns calories and fat does not.

Lean Body Mass Burns Calories And Fat Mass Does Not

Muscle is a constantly changing tissue. It needs to be supplied with energy, it needs to be repaired and rebuilt after minor trauma. In fact, each pound of muscle in your body burns roughly 50 calories a day, even if you don't exercise! These 50 calories are used to maintain the muscle and keep it ready for action.

It may come as no surprise to learn that fat burns virtually no calories. It just kind of hangs out there and stays put. So now we know that fat is inactive tissue while muscle burns calories every day. This is an important point. It would make sense that the more muscle you have, the more calories you will burn each day in an effort to maintain it. This means that you'd burn more of the calories that you ingest and less would be stored as fat. This is the major benefit of resistance training.

As part of the aging process, we start to lose muscle as we enter adulthood. It is estimated that we lose 1% of our lean body mass each year after age 25. Remember, every pound of muscle burns 50 calories a day. Therefore, if you lose 5 pounds of muscle as you enter your mid to late thirties that would be 5 X 50 or 250 calories every day that you once burned but are now storing as body fat. Trust me, this adds up. This is a primary reason why people gain weight as they age, even if their total calorie intake does not increase at all!

With resistance training, you can counter this loss of lean tissue and even increase your lean body mass. In some ways, resistance training is like the fountain of youth. It can roll back the hands of time with regards to your metabolism and lean body mass.

It's also important to realize that when you lose weight without resistance training, you lose both muscle and body fat. This is the body's defense mechanism to prevent its fat stores from dropping too low too fast. After all, we evolved in times of famine and food scarcity. If your fat stores got too low and you hit a famine that would be the end of you. It is estimated that weight loss without resistance exercise results in roughly 50% fat loss and 50% muscle loss. This, as we have just learned, is not good! When you add resistance training to your weight loss plan, you lose a significantly higher amount of fat and a significantly lower amount of muscle, which helps result in permanent weight loss.

Another fear people have concerning weight training is of bulking up and becoming muscle bound, particularly women. First of all, it is not easy to bulk up. Body builders spend a lot of time lifting heavy weights in a highly organized program designed to build muscle. Ask them if it was easy to build all of that muscle and they will tell you "Hell no!". The type of weight training program that I advocate here is to enhance weight loss and general health and fitness, the goal is not to build large amounts of muscle. You will notice increased strength and muscle definition for sure but not large increases in muscle mass. You will be using lighter weights and higher repetitions to help build lean, toned physiques. Women also don't need to worry about bulking up because they generally lack the levels of testosterone necessary for that type of growth.

Frequency And Sample Programs

How many days a week do you need to lift weights? A minimum of 2 and a maximum of 3. It is important to not workout with weights two days in a row. The body needs rest to repair the muscles you use. Therefore, workout on non-consecutive days such as Monday, Wednesday, Friday or Tuesday, Thursday and Saturday. Now I will provide a sample program for men and for women. These are programs designed to enhance weight loss and they can be done quickly; in about 20-30 minutes. Each of these exercises will be illustrated in the next chapter.

Sample Programs
Men

Bench Press	3 sets of 10
1-Arm Row	3 sets of 10
Front Raise	3 sets of 10
Bicep Curl	3 sets of 10
1-Handed Overhead Press	3 sets of 10
Standing Squats	3 sets of 10
Abdominal Crunches	3 sets of 10

Women

Assisted Squats	3 sets of 15
Inner Thigh Lifts	50 (each side)
Standing Side Raise	25 (each side)
Bench Press	3 sets of 15
1-Arm Row	3 sets of 15
Front Raise	3 sets of 15
Bicep Curl	3 sets of 15
Kick back	3 sets of 15
Abdominal Crunches	3 sets of 10

Why is the men's program different than the women's? Most of the men I've trained have the goal of adding a little muscle mass in addition to losing weight. For this reason, the repetitions for their exercises are a little lower and the weights that they use to perform their exercises are significantly higher. This will help them attain their goals. Most of the women I've trained are not at all interested in building large amounts of muscle, they just want to tone up and look tighter. The program for women reflects these goals.

What Weights Should I Use?

This is a very difficult question to address in a book because each person is at a different level of strength and fitness when I first meet them. I've roughly broken it down into 3 classes and then given examples of starting weights. Remember, this is a rough estimate. Your weights will depend on your own subjective view of how hard you are working. Similar to the cardiovascular training guidelines, on a scale from 1 to 10 you should feel like a 7 or 8 on your last set. This is not a maximal effort but no stroll through the park either!

Men Beginner*

Bench Press	8 lb dumbbells
1-Arm Row	8 lb dumbbell
Front Raise	5 lb dumbbells
Bicep Curl	8 lb dumbbells
1-Handed Overhead Press	5 lb dumbbell
Standing Squats	Body Weight

Start with these weights if you have never lifted weights before.

Men Intermediate*

Bench Press	15-20 lb dumbbells
1-Arm Row	15-20 lb dumbbell
Front Raise	8-10 lb dumbbells
Bicep Curl	15 lb dumbbells
1-Handed Overhead Press	8 lb dumbbell
Standing Squats	10 lb dumbbells

Start with these weights if you have some experience with these exercises and weight training in general but have not been lifting consistently.

Men Advanced*

Bench Press	25-30 lb dumbbells
1-Arm Row	25-30 lb dumbbell
Front Raise	12-15 lb dumbbells
Bicep Curl	20-25 lb dumbbells
1-Handed Overhead Press	10-12 lb dumbbell
Standing Squats	15-20 lb dumbbells

Start with these weights if you have been lifting consistently for 2 years or more. These weights may seem low, I'll explain later.

Female Beginner*

Squats	Assisted
Inner Thigh Lift	Body Weight
Standing Side Raise	Body Weight
Bench Press	5 lb dumbbells
1-Arm Row	5 lb dumbbell
Front Raise	3 lb dumbbells
Bicep Curl	5 lb dumbbells
Triceps Kickback	5 lb dumbbell

Start with these weights if you have never lifted weights before.

Female Intermediate*

Squats	Body Weight
Inner Thigh Lift	Body Weight
Standing Side Raise	Body Weight
Bench Press	8 lb dumbbells
1-Arm Row	8 lb dumbbell
Front Raise	5 lb dumbbells
Bicep Curl	8 lb dumbbells
Triceps Kickback	5 lb dumbbell

Start with these weights if you have been lifting for a few months but inconsistently.

<u>Female Advanced*</u>

Squats	5-8 lb dumbbells
Inner Thigh Lift	Body Weight
Standing Side Raise	Body Weight
Bench Press	10 lb dumbbells
1-Arm Row	10 lb dumbbell
Front Raise	6-8 lb dumbbells
Bicep Curl	10 lb dumbbells
Triceps Kickback	8 lb dumbbell

Start with theses weights if you have been lifting consistently for 12 months or more.

Why Are These Weights So Low?

This is a program that is designed to enhance weight loss. It is not designed to build large amounts of muscle or strength. Remember, 50% of your weight loss results will come from dietary change, 30% from cardiovascular exercise and 20% from resistance training. Since most people are really busy and don't have unlimited time to devote to their fitness, these programs cover the bases for resistance training in the shortest time possible. By all means, if you have the time and interest and prefer a more detailed weight training program feel free! But for the goal of weight loss, more extensive programs are not really necessary.

Perform the program with 25 seconds rest in between sets and no rest in between exercises. Wear a watch and time this! There are two ways to get a response from your muscles. You can use heavy weights and take long rests (optimal for body building and higher levels of strength and muscle mass) or you can use lighter weights with shorter rests (optimal for toning and weight loss). I choose the latter for my clients because; 1) They don't have much time and working out this way speeds up the workout. 2) In my experience, lighter weights decrease the risk of injury. Here is an example of a sequence of exercises with the appropriate rest intervals:

Bench Press 1st Set Of 15
--25 Second Rest--
2nd Set Of 15
--25 Second Rest--
3rd Set Of 15
--No Rest—
1-Arm Row 1st Set Of 15
--25 Second Rest—
2nd Set Of 15
--25 Second Rest--
3rd Set Of 15
--No Rest--
Front Raise 1st Set Of 15
--25 Second Rest--
Etc

I would recommend that if at all possible, you do your resistance training at home. Invest in a simple bench and some adjustable dumbbells. Women can buy individual sets of dumbbells; 3lb, 5lb and 8lb are all you'll need. Men can pick up adjustable dumbbells. A set that can take you from 5-30 pounds should do it. You may want to purchase an inexpensive flat bench to help with some of the weight exercises. This equipment won't cost you much and the routines will typically take only 20-25 minutes to do. This is probably less time than it takes to drive to and from the gym and change your clothes.

What About Progression?

For women, whatever level you are, start the weight exercises with 3 sets of 12 repetitions. Slowly increase to 3 sets of 15 repetitions. When this becomes less of a challenge, increase your weight by a few pounds and drop back down to 3 sets of 12. This is called a double progression program.

It is the same idea for men, but start at 3 sets of 8 and work your way up to 3 sets of 10. When this becomes easy, increase the weights by a few pounds and drop back down to 3 sets of 8 repetitions. Take your time increasing your repetitions and weights, this is not a race. Only increase a few repetitions per week.

Your muscles will begin to get used to the challenges that these exercises present and will ultimately stop reacting and growing. For this reason, after 6-8 weeks, it's a good idea to switch up your exercises in order to keep your muscles guessing. For example, for men switch to the following program:

Chest Fly
Overhead Press
Military Press
Concentration Curls
Triceps Kickbacks
Lunges

Here is a second program for women as well:

Plie Squats
Standing Inner Thigh Lifts
Side V's
Chest Fly
Overhead Press
Military Press
Hammer Curls
Overhead Triceps Press

Most of these exercises are really basic. However, if you feel intimidated or unsure, consider hiring a personal trainer for a session or two. It's a great investment to ensure that you are doing the exercises properly. I recommend that you hire a trainer with a degree in exercise science and at least one nationally recognized certification such as ACE (The American Council on Exercise) or ACSM (The American College of Sports Medicine). Remember, although not as important as your diet and your cardio, it is absolutely essential that you fit in at least two and preferably three 20-30 minute weight training sessions a week in order to hit your weight loss goals.

ACTION STEPS FOR THIS CHAPTER

1) Realize the important role of resistance training in the weight loss game.
2) Hit the weights at least twice a week, preferably 3 times a week.
3) Slowly increase your repetitions and your weights. You don't want to simply repeat the same workout over and over. You need to keep your muscles guessing.
4) For the same reason, switch your exercises every 6-8 weeks.
5) If all this seems too intimidating, consider hiring a personal trainer for a session or 2 to get you started.
6) If at all possible, pick up some dumbbells and do your training at home. It will be much easier to fit it in if you don't have to go to the gym to do it.

Chapter 8: *Guide To Resistance Training Exercises*
Bench Press

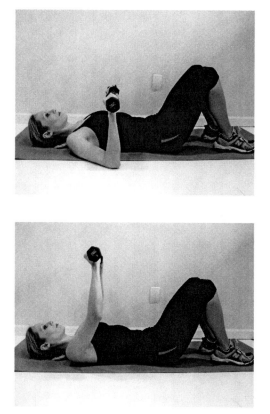

Targets: Chest and Triceps
1) Lie on bench or floor with your back flat and your feet on the floor.
2) Hold dumbbells at the sides of your chest along the line of your sternum (breast plate).
3) Lift dumbbells toward the ceiling.*
4) Slowly return to starting position.

*With this exercise and all others, exhale during the active phase of the exercise, when you are working against gravity. Inhale when you are working with gravity in the passive phase of the exercise. Don't hold your breath! Holding your breath may cause your blood pressure to rise to a dangerous level.

1-Arm Row

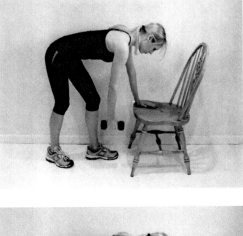

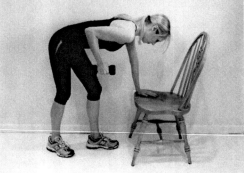

Targets: Back
1) With your left arm on a bench or chair, hold a dumbbell in your right hand.
2) Let your arm hang directly down in front of your shoulder.
3) Slowly pull the dumbbell up toward your chest.
4) Slowly lower the dumbbell to starting position.
5) Keep your back flat and centered over the bench. Your elbow should be tight against your ribcage as you lift and lower the dumbbell.
6) Alternate sets between your right and left hand.

Front Raise

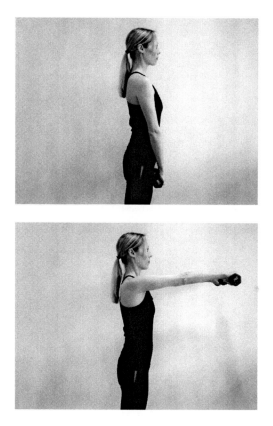

Targets: Shoulders
1) Stand up straight with your feet shoulder width apart.
2) Hold dumbbells directly in front of you with your palms facing your thighs.
3) Slowly raise dumbbells to shoulder level (no higher).
4) Slowly lower to starting position.

Bicep Curl

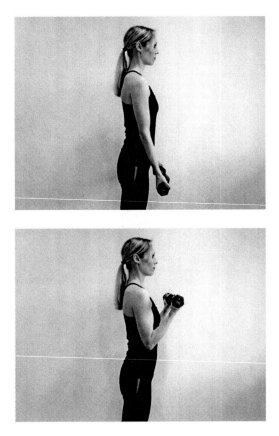

Targets: Biceps
1) Stand with your feet shoulder width apart and your knees slightly bent.
2) Hold dumbbells with your arms at your sides and your palms facing forward.
3) Keep your shoulders still and slowly bend your elbows to raise dumbbells by just moving your forearms.
4) Slowly return to starting position.

1-Handed Overhead Triceps Press

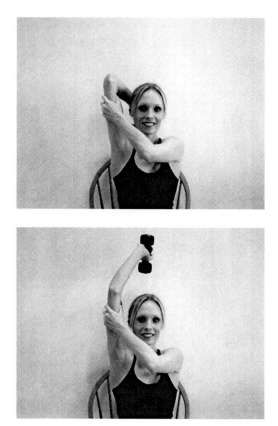

Targets: Triceps
1) Grasp a dumbbell with your right hand behind your head with your elbow bent.
2) Keep your upper arm fixed from shoulder to elbow.
3) Raise the dumbbell toward the ceiling until your arm is straight.
4) Slowly return to starting position.
5) Alternate sets with right and left hand.

Standing Squats

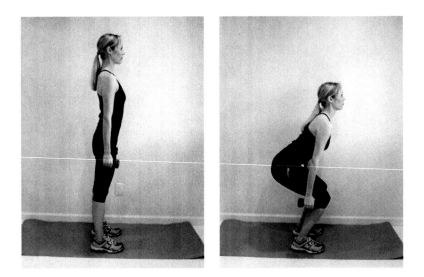

Targets: Legs
1) Stand upright with your feet shoulder width apart.
2) Hold dumbbells at your sides.
3) Bend your knees until your thighs are almost parallel to the ground.
4) Slowly return to starting position.
5) Don't let your knees cross the plane of your toes.

Abdominal Crunches

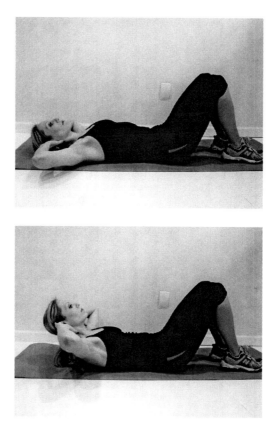

Targets: Stomach (abdominals)
1) Lie on your back with your knees bent and your feet flat on the ground.
2) Put your hands behind your head with your elbows pointing outward.
3) Curl your body upward toward your thighs until your trunk reaches a 45° angle with the floor.
4) Slowly lower to starting position.
5) Keep your feet on the floor at all times.

Assisted Squats

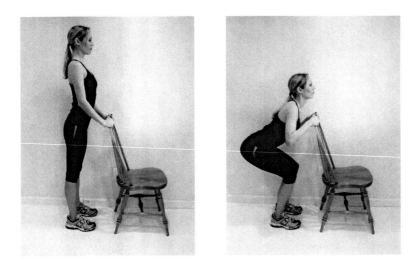

Targets: Legs
1) Stand in front of a pole or a sturdy chair with your feet shoulder width apart.
2) Slowly bend your knees until your thighs are almost parallel to the floor.
3) Hold onto a pole or chair for balance only. Don't use the chair to pull yourself up. Your weight should be on your feet so your legs do the work.
4) Slowly rise to starting position.
5) Make sure your knees don't cross the plane of your toes. This puts unnecessary strain on your knee joint.

Inner Thigh Lift

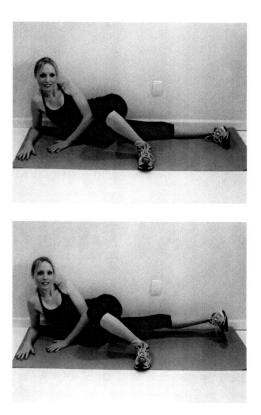

Targets: Inside of thigh
1) Lay on your right side with your right leg straight and your left leg bent over your right leg.
2) Keeping your right leg completely straight, raise it up toward the ceiling.
3) Slowly lower to starting position.
4) Repeat on your left side.

Standing Side Raise

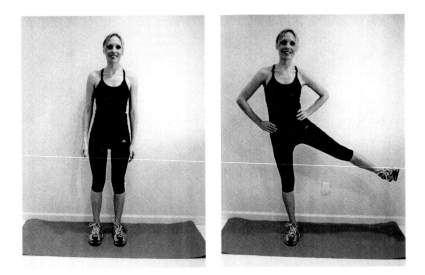

Targets: Outer thigh
1) Stand up straight and lean your right hand against a wall or pole for balance if necessary.
2) Raise your left leg until it is nearly parallel to the floor.
3) Slowly return to starting position.
4) Alternate sets between your left and right legs.

Triceps Kickback

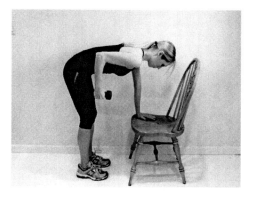

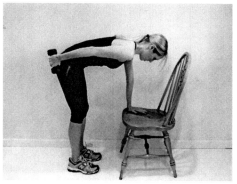

Targets: Triceps
1) Hold a dumbbell in your right hand.
2) Bend at your waist and rest your left hand on a bench or chair.
3) Your back should be parallel to the floor.
4) Raise your elbow up to the level of your ribcage and keep your arm close to your body.
5) Extend the dumbbell back until your arm is straight, keeping your upper arm motionless. Only your forearm should be moving.
6) Slowly return to starting position.
7) Alternate sets between your left and right arm.

Chest Fly

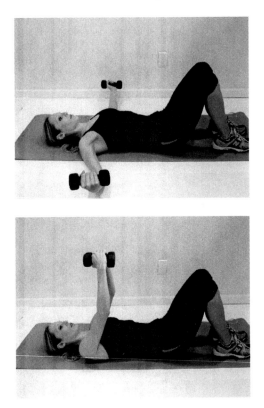

Targets: Chest
1) Lie on floor or a bench.
2) Grasp a pair of dumbbells and hold them above your chest with your palms facing one another.
3) With elbows slightly bent, lower your arms until they are slightly above your shoulders.
4) Keep the weights in line with your breast bone.
5) Slowly return to starting position.

Overhead Press

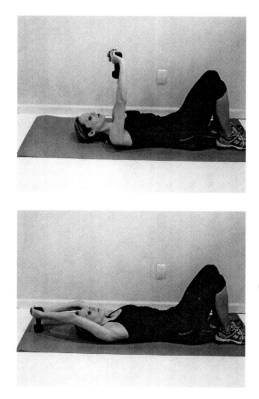

Targets: Back
1) Lie on floor or bench (bend knees if on floor).
2) Hold a dumbbell between your thumb and fore-finger of both hands letting it lay perpendicularly above your chest.
3) With your arms straight, extend the dumbbell behind your head until it almost reaches the bench or floor.
4) Slowly bring back to starting position.

Military Press

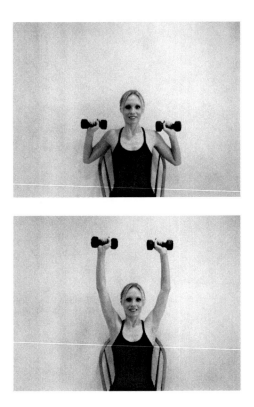

Targets: Shoulder
1) Sit on a chair or bench with your feet flat on the floor.
2) Hold dumbbells at shoulder height with your palms facing forward.
3) Raise the dumbbells toward the ceiling keeping them lined up with your ears.
4) Slowly lower the dumbbells back to starting position.

Concentration Curls

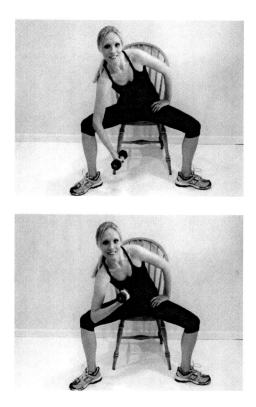

Targets: Biceps
1) Sit on a chair or bench with your legs spread wide apart.
2) Hold a dumbbell with your arm pressed against your inner thigh.
3) Curl the weight up toward your chin.
4) Slowly lower to starting position.
5) Alternate sets between your right and left side.

Lunge

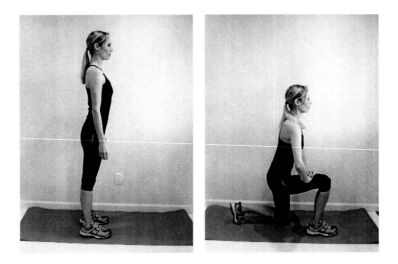

Targets: Legs
1) Stand with your feet shoulder width apart.
2) Slowly step forward with your right leg and drop your left knee almost to the ground. Rest your hands on your right thigh.
3) Make sure your knee does not cross the plane of your toes.
4) Slowly return to starting position.
5) Alternate sets between your right and left leg.

Plie Squats

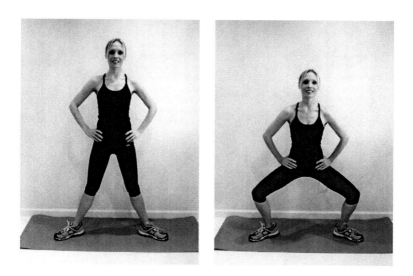

Targets: Legs
1) Stand with your feet spread widely apart and your toes pointing outward.
2) Bend down at the knee until your thighs are almost parallel to the floor.
3) Slowly return to starting position.

Standing Inner Thigh Lifts

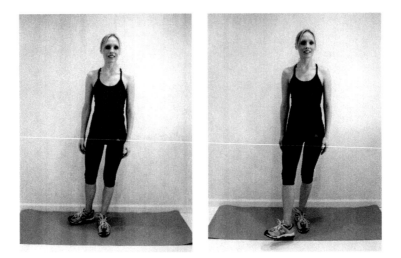

Targets: Inner thigh
1) Stand up straight and lean against a pole or wall for balance, if necessary.
2) Point the toes of your right foot outward so you form a right angle with your left foot.
3) Move leg forward 1-2 feet.
4) Slowly return to starting position.
5) Alternate sets between both legs.

Side V's

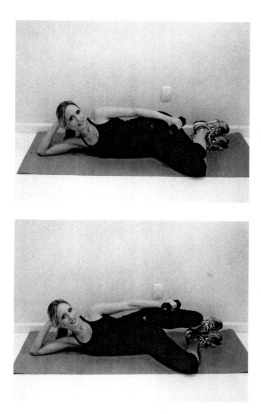

Targets: Outer thigh
1) Lay down on your right side with your knees bent and your feet together.
2) Hold a dumbbell on your left thigh midway between your knee and hip.
3) Slowly open your legs apart, keeping your feet together at all times.
4) Slowly return to starting position.
5) Alternate sets between both legs.

Hammer Curls

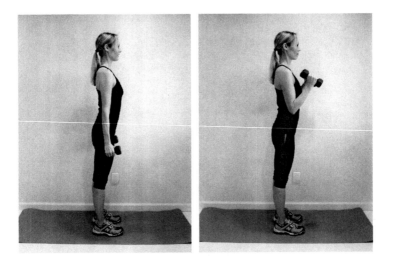

Targets: Bicep
1) Stand with your feet shoulder width apart and knees slightly bent.
2) Hold dumbbells with your arms at your sides and your palms facing one another.
3) Keep shoulders still and slowly bend your elbows to raise dumbbells by just moving your forearm.
4) Slowly return to starting position.

Chapter 9

Lifestyle Factors: The Icing On The Cake

OK, so we've covered the big 3 components of the program; diet, cardio and resistance training, now it's time for the icing on the cake. Following are lifestyle and behavioral factors that will go a long way in helping along the weight loss process.

#1 Write Down What You Eat And Your Daily Cardio Minutes.

Keeping a record of your diet and cardio is a valuable tool to help you gauge your progress. It is also accountability! Knowing that you have to answer to someone, even if it is yourself, helps you to make better choices consistently.

In fact, I recently attended an obesity symposium at Harvard Medical School where a researcher there told an interesting story. This particular scientist had designed a study to examine the effects of 2 different diets on weight loss, a low fat diet and a low carbohydrate diet. The idea was to separate the subjects into 2 groups, one group would follow the low fat diet and the other would follow the low carb diet for several months and then the amount of weight lost would be compared between the 2 groups. In an effort to make sure that the 2 groups were similar in their baseline diets prior to entering the study, the participants were told to simply write down everything that they ate for a period of 2 weeks. They were instructed not to change anything about their diet, just to write it down. Would you believe that every single participant lost weight in these 2 weeks, by doing nothing more than writing down what they ate?

I have my clients write down what they eat for at least a few months. It is invaluable for giving them a sense of control over their food selections. It sounds like an inconvenience, but in actuality it takes just 30 seconds after each meal; just 1.5 minutes a day to greatly help you toward your weight loss goals. Well worth the investment!!! Again, this won't need to go on forever but do it for the first few months. A simple pocket sized memo book is all you will need. Simply write the date on top of the page and then fill in your carbohydrate, fat and protein selection for breakfast, lunch and dinner. See the sample on the following page.

It's equally important to document your cardiovascular exercise. How else will you be able to tell with certainty if you have hit your weekly goal of cardio minutes? Furthermore, if you have a week or two where your weight loss has slowed, it is very easy to see which part of your program was responsible for the plateau if you've kept records of your diet and cardio.

Monday July 18th   **Cardio Minutes:** 45 minutes

Breakfast: Protein: Low fat plain yogurt

           Carbohydrate: Strawberries and blueberries

           Fat: Peanut butter

Lunch: Protein: Tuna fish

           Carbohydrate: Salad vegetables

           Fat: Olive oil based dressing

Dinner: Protein: Chicken breast

           Carbohydrate: Brown rice, vegetable stir-fry

           Fat: Canola oil used in stir fry

#2 No Eating After 8:00 PM

This is a really important lifestyle change if you want to be successful in the weight loss game. I don't think anyone knows for certain why this works but in my experience it totally does.

Some believe that our metabolism slows down significantly in the evening and since we're not burning many calories, more of what we eat turns to fat. I don't know if I believe that entirely, but it may be true. I think this one is important because if you don't eat anything after 8:00 pm, you simply are decreasing your calories for the day. Furthermore, the 300, 400 or even 800 calories you're taking in after dinner in front of the television are not, shall we say, the most nutritious!

I have had clients who were exercising well and following the dietary plan well but lost little weight until they implemented this rule. I can add a little story from my own personal experience. Growing up, I had the exact opposite problem that my clients hire me to help them solve. I could not gain weight for the life of me. You could count my ribs- I was that skinny. I was tired of looking so emaciated as I got into high school and started eating all the time. Nothing happened! I got a job at a bake shop and literally ate bread, cookies and anything else for 5 or 6 hours after school. Unbelievably, I still would not gain a pound. My metabolism just seemed to eat up whatever I threw at it.

I graduated high school and went off to college as thin as ever. A fraternity brother told me that one of his buddies back home had the same problem and he finally gained weight by eating 2 peanut butter sandwiches right before bed. Well I tried it and gained 30 lbs in 4 months! I tell you this story to make the following point; if eating food late at night finally put weight on a young kid with a super high metabolism, what will it do to someone who has a slow metabolism? You guessed it, nothing good. No eating after 8:00 PM.

Do your very best with this one. I know it can be difficult. People are in the habit of making dinner reservations at 8 or 9 or even 10 PM on the weekends. This must change. Make your reservations a little earlier. Have dinner first on your own and then meet up socially for a movie or something else. You need to learn that your lifestyle habits are the major reason why you have gained weight in the first place. If you don't change them you'll be stuck in the same situation for sure.

#3 Drink 8 Glasses Of Water A Day

Everyone who is interested in losing weight has heard this one a million times. Drink 8 glasses of water a day. There are a variety of reasons why this is so helpful; some are proven, some are not.

1) The body needs water to break down fat. The theory here is that the breakdown of body fat is a hydrolysis reaction (one that requires water). If you are dehydrated, this process is slowed down and optimal fat loss is not achieved. I don't know how much hard evidence there is for this one, but I thought I'd throw it out as a possibility.

2) Water acts as a satiety factor. I have seen studies that show those who drink a glass or 2 of water before a meal tend to eat less than those who do not.

3) Take away the goal of weight loss and it is still a very important to drink enough water. First,

dehydration can make you feel tired, irritable and less productive in all you do. Secondly, when you are dehydrated, exercise is a lot harder and less enjoyable.

A couple of notes on the water intake. Do your very best to sip water throughout the day instead of chugging 2 or 3 glasses at once when you realize you're behind on your water requirement. This is to avoid having to run to the bathroom often, which is the biggest complaint that I get on this one.

Another thing to realize is that any sugar or caffeine containing beverage does not count toward your 8 glasses a day. Sugar and caffeine are diuretics that direct the body to excrete water. Not what we are trying to accomplish! A general rule is to add a cup of water to your requirement for every cup of coffee or tea you consume. For example, if you have 2 cups of coffee a day, your total has jumped from 8 glasses to 10.

Most of us walk around dehydrated all the time and don't even know it. When you are well hydrated you'll feel better and have more energy. Do your very best with this one!

Specifics On Beverages
Fruit Juices-No Good; Sugar
Diet Soda-No Good; Caffeine
Coffee/Tea-No Good; Caffeine
Club Soda/Sparkling Water-Good!
Decaf Coffee/Tea-Good But Don't Add Sugar

#4 Easy On The Alcohol

Alcohol has become an area of great interest in the fields of nutrition and medicine in recent years. Too much alcohol is like poison to the body causing a variety of negative health effects such as liver disorders, cancer and vitamin deficiency as seen in alcoholics. However, a moderate amount of alcohol (approximately 1 drink a day) appears to decrease the risk of heart disease, stroke, and diabetes as well as increase overall longevity.

These two facts have put doctors and nutritionists in a difficult position regarding alcohol recommend-dations. On the one hand, we don't want to push alcohol use and risk alcoholism in those genetically prone to this terrible disorder. Yet the potential health benefits of moderate alcohol use are difficult to ignore. I hate to complicate matters further, but here goes;

If you want to lose weight, strictly limit alcohol use, particularly during the main thrust of your weight loss effort (prior to weight maintenance). There are at least 3 reasons why this is important.

1) Alcohol is calorie dense, it contains 7 calories per gram and these are nutritionally empty calories that provide little besides energy. A typical beer has 150 calories, a glass of wine has 85 calories and 1.5 ounces of hard liquor generally has 100 calories. Have 2 or 3 of these a day and trust me, the calories begin to add up.

2) Many theorize that chronic alcohol use decreases your metabolic rate, causing you to burn fewer overall calories. I have not seen much hard scientific evidence of this but I thought I'd throw it out there as a possibility.

3) In my experience and that of my clients, when you have a few drinks and start to get a bit of a buzz, your discipline goes out the window. When you drink, inhibitions of all types are lessened. You begin to think "Why not, you only live once". This causes many otherwise bright people to make bad decisions! After 3 or 4 drinks, the dessert menu becomes harder to resist and the late night fast food/diner stop seems to become all but inevitable!

You don't necessarily have to give up alcohol here. If you have a few drinks a week, say three or less, you'll be fine. If you're drinking every day, this can really slow you down with regards to weight loss.

#5 Limit Sugar-Free Sweeteners

As you have probably noticed, the increase in the prevalence of type 2 diabetes and the popularity of low carbohydrate diets has created a gigantic market for sugar free products. It is now common to see sugar free ice-cream, cookies, candies and protein bars in addition to the all familiar diet soda. The sweeteners used in these products are fairly well tested and overall pretty safe when consumed occasionally. When trying to decrease the sugar content of your diet, it is common to want to load up on the sugar free products to make you feel less deprived.

An occasional diet soda or sugar free candy won't do much harm and can be a real treat. However, don't go overboard with this. Although these products will not raise blood sugar or cause a large release of insulin, they do tend to perpetuate your cravings for sweets and refined carbohydrates. If you get sugar out of your diet, in about 2-3 weeks you won't miss it or crave it at all. If you consistently consume these sugar free products, the cravings never really go away entirely and you'll always be fighting them to one degree or another. This is a problem because any diet where there is a continuing feeling of deprivation will not result in long term weight loss.

Another problem with the non-nutritive sweeteners is something called the cephalic response. If you were to put your favorite food in front of yourself, your eyes would see it, your nose would smell it and your body anticipates you are about to eat it. There is evidence that your body releases digestive enzymes in anticipation of the meal before you even put it in your mouth! The same may be happening with the non-nutritive sweeteners. The body thinks it's getting sugar when you eat these and may release insulin in response. This is exactly what we are trying to limit. There are some studies that show those who eat lots of sugar free items actually gain more weight than those that eat the regular sugar containing products! Limit yourself to at most 1 or 2 diet sodas a week and 1 or 2 sugar free treats per week in order to keep these cravings at bay.

#6 Shoot For At Least 7 Hours Of Sleep Each Night

This is relatively cutting edge research but several well designed studies are pointing to the fact that not sleeping enough can have a negative effect on hormones that dictate appetite and body fat storage (ghrelin and leptin) and can lower your metabolic rate (which dictates how many calories you burn per day). Do your best to get at least 7 hours of sleep each night.

#7 Planned Relapses (AKA Splurge Meals)

No diet needs to be 100% perfect in order to attain your weight loss or overall health goals. I've asked you to change your diet dramatically and to give up foods that you were eating every day and love to eat. Total deprivation of these foods is neither realistic nor necessary. If your diet is 90% on, you will hit your weight loss goals for sure. That means that 10% of the time you can have some fun. Since we eat 3 meals a day for 7 days a week, that's 21 meals per week and 10% of 21 is approximately 2. So for 2 meals a week you can basically ignore everything I've told you about diet and eat exactly what you want. I call these splurge meals or planned relapses.

Did you really think that I'd ask you to give up bread, pasta and dessert forever? We both know that's not going to work. If I did you'd probably hang in there for a few weeks, maybe even a few months but eventually you'd break down and have something from the avoid column and say "This guy is crazy, I can't do this anymore" and pretty much quit. I call these splurge meals a planned relapse because you have total control over them. You plan when you have them and you stop after 2 a week and there is no guilt because you've done nothing wrong. They go in your food log and you get back on track the very next meal.

If you're smart, you'll plan one of these splurge meals on Wednesday and the other one on Saturday so you never have to go more than 3 days without one of your favorite foods you're trying to cut back on. Be creative, if it's pizza that you miss the most have that. If it's a cheeseburger then go for it! No guilt, no worries. Plan them out. If you know you'll be having dinner at a wedding or party, don't even try to be good, make it a splurge meal and have fun with it. The key is control. It all goes in the food log and remember, any two meals you want can be splurge meals but only two a week.

There is only one rule when it comes to splurge meals: Stay away from sugar. If you have sugar even twice a week, there is a really good chance you will start to want it all the time. The reason this dietary plan works so well is that after a couple of weeks, there really is no deprivation. Once your blood sugar stabilizes, you won't crave bread, pasta, rice and sugar. If you are constantly battling cravings for sugar, it will be very hard to stay focused. It sounds unbelievable but it's true: It is easier to give up sugar 100% than 75%.

However, we all like something sweet now and again. There is currently a huge assortment of sugar free treats available. You can find sugar free chocolate, peanut butter cups, ice cream, cookies and even cupcakes. Feel free to enjoy some sugar free treats during or after your splurge meals. They are made with non-nutritive sweeteners and sugar alcohols. Start slowly with them because the sugar alcohols can have a laxative effect in sensitive people and that's no fun for anyone.

<u>ACTION STEPS FOR THIS CHAPTER</u>

1) Keep a log of your diet and cardio minutes.
2) Absolutely no eating after 8:00 PM.
3) Drink 8 glasses of water each day.
4) Keep alcohol containing drinks to 3 or less per week during the weight loss phase.
5) Limit non-nutritive sweeteners to a couple of times a week.
6) Try to get at least 7 hours of sleep each night.
7) Plan 2 splurge meals a week. Feel free to eat anything you want during these meals except for sugar. If you want something sweet after a splurge meal, grab a sugar free treat.

Chapter 10: *30 Days On The Triad*

This chapter contains 30 days of food and exercise logs to help you get started on the program. Remember, record keeping is pivotal to your success!

DAY 1

Date: _____

Breakfast: Protein: _____
　　　　Carbohydrate: _____
　　　　Fat: _____

Lunch: Protein: _____
　　　　Carbohydrate: _____
　　　　Fat: _____

Dinner: Protein: _____
　　　　Carbohydrate: _____
　　　　Fat: _____

Cardio Minutes: _____

Weight Training: Y　N

Weight: _____ lbs

Waist*: _____ inches

Hips**: _____ inches

---

*Measure your waist right at the line of your belly-button
**Measure your hips half-way between your hip joint and your knee joint

DAY 2

Date: _____

Breakfast: Protein: _____

Carbohydrate: _____

Fat: _____

Lunch: Protein: _____

Carbohydrate: _____

Fat: _____

Dinner: Protein: _____

Carbohydrate: _____

Fat: _____

Cardio Minutes: _____

Weight Training: Y   N

DAY 3

Date: _____

Cardio Minutes: _____

Breakfast: Protein: _____

Weight Training: Y   N

Carbohydrate: _____

Fat: _____

Lunch: Protein: _____

Carbohydrate: _____

Fat: _____

Dinner: Protein: _____

Carbohydrate: _____

Fat: _____

DAY 4

Date: _____

Breakfast: Protein: _____

         Carbohydrate: _____

         Fat: _____

Lunch: Protein: _____

        Carbohydrate: _____

        Fat: _____

Dinner: Protein: _____

        Carbohydrate: _____

        Fat: _____

Cardio Minutes: _____

Weight Training: Y   N

DAY 5

Date: _____

Breakfast: Protein: _____

                Carbohydrate: _____

                Fat: _____

Lunch: Protein: _____

              Carbohydrate: _____

              Fat: _____

Dinner: Protein: _____

              Carbohydrate: _____

              Fat: _____

Cardio Minutes: _____

Weight Training: Y   N

DAY 6

Date: _____   **Cardio Minutes:** _____

Breakfast: Protein: _____   **Weight Training:** Y   N

Carbohydrate: _____

Fat: _____

Lunch: Protein: _____

Carbohydrate: _____

Fat: _____

Dinner: Protein: _____

Carbohydrate: _____

Fat: _____

DAY 7

Date: _____

Cardio Minutes: _____

Breakfast: Protein: _____

Carbohydrate: _____

Fat: _____

Weight Training: Y   N

Weight: _____ lbs

Lunch: Protein: _____

Carbohydrate: _____

Fat: _____

Dinner: Protein: _____

Carbohydrate: _____

Fat: _____

DAY 8

Date: _____   **Cardio Minutes:** _____

Breakfast: Protein: _____   **Weight Training:** Y   N

   Carbohydrate: _____

   Fat: _____

Lunch: Protein: _____

   Carbohydrate: _____

   Fat: _____

Dinner: Protein: _____

   Carbohydrate: _____

   Fat: _____

DAY 9

Date: _____

Breakfast: Protein: _____
            Carbohydrate: _____
            Fat: _____

Lunch: Protein: _____
         Carbohydrate: _____
         Fat: _____

Dinner: Protein: _____
          Carbohydrate: _____
          Fat: _____

Cardio Minutes: _____

Weight Training: Y   N

DAY 10

Date: _____

Breakfast: Protein: _____
              Carbohydrate: _____
              Fat: _____

Lunch: Protein: _____
          Carbohydrate: _____
          Fat: _____

Dinner: Protein: _____
           Carbohydrate: _____
           Fat: _____

Cardio Minutes: _____

Weight Training: Y   N

DAY 11

Date: _____

Breakfast: Protein: _____

Carbohydrate: _____

Fat: _____

Lunch: Protein: _____

Carbohydrate: _____

Fat: _____

Dinner: Protein: _____

Carbohydrate: _____

Fat: _____

Cardio Minutes: _____

Weight Training: Y   N

DAY 12

Date: _____

Breakfast: Protein: _____

           Carbohydrate: _____

           Fat: _____

Lunch: Protein: _____

        Carbohydrate: _____

        Fat: _____

Dinner: Protein: _____

        Carbohydrate: _____

        Fat: _____

Cardio Minutes: _____

Weight Training: Y   N

DAY 13

Date: _____   **Cardio Minutes:** _____

Breakfast: Protein: _____   **Weight Training:** Y   N

Carbohydrate: _____

Fat: _____

Lunch: Protein: _____

Carbohydrate: _____

Fat: _____

Dinner: Protein: _____

Carbohydrate: _____

Fat: _____

DAY 14

Date: _____

Breakfast: Protein: _____

              Carbohydrate: _____

              Fat: _____

Lunch: Protein: _____

         Carbohydrate: _____

         Fat: _____

Dinner: Protein: _____

         Carbohydrate: _____

         Fat: _____

Cardio Minutes: _____

Weight Training: Y   N

Weight: _____ lbs

DAY 15

Date: _____

Cardio Minutes: _____

Breakfast: Protein: _____

Weight Training: Y   N

Carbohydrate: _____

Fat: _____

Lunch: Protein: _____

Carbohydrate: _____

Fat: _____

Dinner: Protein: _____

Carbohydrate: _____

Fat: _____

DAY 16

Date: _____

Cardio Minutes: _____

Breakfast: Protein: _____

Weight Training: Y   N

Carbohydrate: _____

Fat: _____

Lunch: Protein: _____

Carbohydrate: _____

Fat: _____

Dinner: Protein: _____

Carbohydrate: _____

Fat: _____

DAY 17

Date: _____

Cardio Minutes: _____

Breakfast: Protein: _____

Weight Training: Y   N

Carbohydrate: _____

Fat: _____

Lunch: Protein: _____

Carbohydrate: _____

Fat: _____

Dinner: Protein: _____

Carbohydrate: _____

Fat: _____

DAY 18

Date: _____

Cardio Minutes: _____

Breakfast: Protein: _____

Weight Training: Y   N

Carbohydrate: _____

Fat: _____

Lunch: Protein: _____

Carbohydrate: _____

Fat: _____

Dinner: Protein: _____

Carbohydrate: _____

Fat: _____

DAY 19

Date: _____

Cardio Minutes: _____

Breakfast: Protein: _____

Weight Training: Y   N

Carbohydrate: _____

Fat: _____

Lunch: Protein: _____

Carbohydrate: _____

Fat: _____

Dinner: Protein: _____

Carbohydrate: _____

Fat: _____

DAY 20

Date: _____

Breakfast: Protein: _____

            Carbohydrate: _____

            Fat: _____

Lunch: Protein: _____

            Carbohydrate: _____

            Fat: _____

Dinner: Protein: _____

            Carbohydrate: _____

            Fat: _____

Cardio Minutes: _____

Weight Training: Y   N

DAY 21

Date: _____

Breakfast: Protein: _____

Carbohydrate: _____

Fat: _____

Lunch: Protein: _____

Carbohydrate: _____

Fat: _____

Dinner: Protein: _____

Carbohydrate: _____

Fat: _____

Cardio Minutes: _____

Weight Training: Y   N

Weight: _____ lbs

DAY 22

Date: _____

Cardio Minutes: _____

Breakfast: Protein: _____

Weight Training: Y   N

Carbohydrate: _____

Fat: _____

Lunch: Protein: _____

Carbohydrate: _____

Fat: _____

Dinner: Protein: _____

Carbohydrate: _____

Fat: _____

DAY 23

Date: _____

Breakfast: Protein: _____
　　　　　　Carbohydrate: _____
　　　　　　Fat: _____

Lunch: Protein: _____
　　　　Carbohydrate: _____
　　　　Fat: _____

Dinner: Protein: _____
　　　　　Carbohydrate: _____
　　　　　Fat: _____

Cardio Minutes: _____

Weight Training: Y　N

DAY 24

Date: _____

Breakfast: Protein: _____

            Carbohydrate: _____

            Fat: _____

Lunch: Protein: _____

         Carbohydrate: _____

         Fat: _____

Dinner: Protein: _____

          Carbohydrate: _____

          Fat: _____

Cardio Minutes: _____

Weight Training: Y   N

DAY 25

Date: _____

Cardio Minutes: _____

Breakfast: Protein: _____

Weight Training: Y   N

Carbohydrate: _____

Fat: _____

Lunch: Protein: _____

Carbohydrate: _____

Fat: _____

Dinner: Protein: _____

Carbohydrate: _____

Fat: _____

DAY 26

Date: _____

Cardio Minutes: _____

Breakfast: Protein: _____

Weight Training: Y   N

Carbohydrate: _____

Fat: _____

Lunch: Protein: _____

Carbohydrate: _____

Fat: _____

Dinner: Protein: _____

Carbohydrate: _____

Fat: _____

DAY 27

Date: _____   **Cardio Minutes:** _____

Breakfast: Protein: _____   **Weight Training:** Y   N

Carbohydrate: _____

Fat: _____

Lunch: Protein: _____

Carbohydrate: _____

Fat: _____

Dinner: Protein: _____

Carbohydrate: _____

Fat: _____

DAY 28

Date: _____

Breakfast: Protein: _____
　　　　Carbohydrate: _____
　　　　Fat: _____

Lunch: Protein: _____
　　　Carbohydrate: _____
　　　Fat: _____

Dinner: Protein: _____
　　　Carbohydrate: _____
　　　Fat: _____

Cardio Minutes: _____

Weight Training: Y　　N

Weight: _____ lbs

DAY 29

Date: _____

Breakfast: Protein: _____

Carbohydrate: _____

Fat: _____

Lunch: Protein: _____

Carbohydrate: _____

Fat: _____

Dinner: Protein: _____

Carbohydrate: _____

Fat: _____

Cardio Minutes: _____

Weight Training: Y   N

DAY 30

Date: _____

Breakfast: Protein: _____

Carbohydrate: _____

Fat: _____

Lunch: Protein: _____

Carbohydrate: _____

Fat: _____

Dinner: Protein: _____

Carbohydrate: _____

Fat: _____

Cardio Minutes: _____

Weight Training: Y   N

Weight: _____ lbs

Waist*: ____ inches

Hips:** ____ inches

*Measure your waist right at the line of your belly-button
**Measure your hips half-way between your hip joint and your knee joint

Chapter 11

Life On The Triad

OK, so you've finished the book. I've thrown a lot at you and I'm sure your head is spinning! You should feel optimistic because you are about to make some great changes that will influence just about every aspect of your life. Congrats for taking the first important step.

One last piece of advice; slow and steady wins the race. Very few people can just adopt all of these lifestyle changes right away. Some get their cardio and diet down but have trouble with the weight training. Maybe getting the cardio in will be your greatest challenge.

The weight loss process has a lot of ups and downs, good weeks and bad weeks. The key to success is not to be perfect in following the program but rather lies in picking yourself up when you fall down. Persistence is the key to weight loss but remember this is not rocket science. This program works and you can make it work for you. Remember, I've just given you the "gold standard" for weight loss, everything you can do to lose weight effectively and permanently. You'll also lose weight on the "silver" or "bronze" standard but just a bit more slowly. In other words, if you are only able to do ¾ of what I'm asking you to do, you'll still get results, just more slowly.

Keep taking baby steps- every week strive to be a little more diligent about one aspect of the program that is giving you trouble. Before you know it you'll be there. Good luck!!!

How Fast Will I Lose The Weight?

You need to understand that one pound of fat is a lot of calories, 3500 in fact. To lose one pound of fat in a week, you'd have to create a caloric deficit of 500 calories every day. That is either eat 500 fewer calories or exercise away 500 calories. This is easier said than done.

We live in a world where people expect fast results. You can get a meal at a fast food restaurant in 2 minutes. You get money from an ATM instantaneously. Our bodies don't work quite the same way. Most experts will tell you that the human body can lose at most 2 pounds of fat in a week. People who claim they lost 8 pounds in a week on a low carbohydrate diet or 7 pounds a week on a liquid diet are confused. They indeed may have lost 8 pounds of weight in a week, but they certainly didn't lose 8 pounds of fat in a week. The majority of this quick weight loss is water and lean body mass.

For my male clients, 2 pounds of fat loss in a week is not uncommon. A good average is 1 pound a week. Women have it a bit tougher, ¾ of a pound a week on average is great. Three-quarters of a pound a week may not sound like much but that's 36 pounds in a year and will result in permanent weight loss since we are sparing lean tissue. Remember to always look to the average. You may lose a lot of weight in one week, lose nothing in the next week and then even gain a pound in the following week. Always look at the average. As long as you are at or above ¾ of a pound a week, the program is working.

Don't get too wrapped up on weight. Remember, you are adding muscle while you are losing fat. The scale will reflect this. I suggest that you weigh yourself one time a week, the same day every week, first thing in the morning without any clothes on at all.

Make sure at least 2 days have passed since your last splurge meal before you weigh yourself. The reason for this is that consuming extra salt, alcohol or white flour can cause you to retain a few pounds of water for a couple of days. Ladies, also keep in mind that during that time of the month you can also retain a few pounds of water so don't freak out if the scale goes up a bit around this time every month.

The main indicator of how you are doing with your weight loss efforts will be how your clothes fit you. If you want a more formal gauge of progress, take measurements of your waist (right at the line of your belly-button) and your hips (half-way between your hip joint and your knee joint). Even better, get your body fat tested every few months. Most trainers and nutritionists can do this for you for a small fee. Always keep in mind that the scale is not the whole story. It will not be able to tell you about your changing body composition.

Maintenance After You Have Hit Your Goal Weight

You need to realize that this is not a temporary weight loss diet or exercise plan. These changes need to become a way of life and while you don't need to be as strict during maintenance, the last thing you want to do is revert back to the old habits that caused you to gain weight in the first place. Having said that, once you have hit your goal weight, you are not going to have to be quite as strict with your diet and cardiovascular exercise program.

Maintenance of weight lost is highly subjective; it will be different for each person. Continue with your weight training at least twice a week in order to maintain and add to your muscle mass. Once you are happy with your weight, you can generally add another splurge meal and decrease your cardio minutes by about one third. So if you are a guy doing 150 minutes of cardio a week, you can maintain your weight loss with about 100 minutes a week. If you are a gal doing 250 minutes of cardio a week you can maintain your weight by doing about 170 minutes a week. You may be able to get away with more or less depending on your situation.

By the time most of my clients hit the point of maintenance, they have a really good grasp of the program and how to make it work for them. Generally, it is trial and error; if you notice you have gained a pound or 2 back, maybe adjust your cardio or splurge meal frequency to strike a balance. The good news is that at this point, it is all under your control. You know what to do to lose weight!

Congratulations!!!

<u>SUMMARY</u>

1) Combine **Best Choices** of Fat, Protein and Carbohydrate at each and every meal or snack.
2) Complete the required number of cardio minutes at the proper intensity. This number will be specific for you but the average number for women is 250 minutes a week and for men it is 150 minutes per week.
3) Complete at least 2 sessions of resistance training per week in order to maintain and add to your metabolically active lean body mass.
4) Keep a log of your diet and cardio minutes.
5) No eating after 8:00 PM.
6) If you drink, limit alcoholic beverages to 3 per week, at least until you hit your goal weight.
7) Drink 8 glasses of water per day.
8) Feel free to take 2 splurge meals a week to keep you honest for the long term.

<u>ACTION STEPS FOR THIS CHAPTER</u>

1) Have realistic weight loss goals: 1 pound a week for men and ¾ of a pound a week for women.

2) Weigh yourself once a week, first thing in the morning at least 2 days after your last splurge meal. Record the number in your log.

3) Don't get too wrapped up on the scale. Remember, you will be adding small amounts of muscle while decreasing your body fat and the scale will reflect this. Go instead with how your clothes are fitting you, your circumference measurements or your body fat measurement.

4) Once you hit your goal weight, feel free to go on maintenance. This is generally one extra splurge meal a week and about 30% less cardio. But it is different for every person and trial and error will help you figure out your own personal maintenance plan.

CPSIA information can be obtained at www.ICGtesting.com
Printed in the USA
LVOW032031160911

246543LV00006B/131/P